ABC OF
ANTENATAL CARE

Fourth edition

GEOFFREY CHAMBERLAIN

Professor Emeritus, Department of Obstetrics and Gynaecology,
St George's Hospital Medical School, London and
Consultant Obstetrician, Singleton Hospital, Swansea

and

MARGERY MORGAN

Consultant Obstetrician and Gynaecologist, Singleton Hospital, Swansea

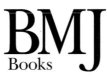

BMJ
Books

First published in 1992
Second edition 1994
Third edition 1997
Fourth edition 2002
by BMJ Books, BMA House, Tavistock Square,
London WC1H 9JR

www.bmjbooks.com

British Library Cataloguing in Publication Data
A catalogue record for this book is available from the British Library

ISBN 0-7279-1692-0

Cover image depicts body contour map of
a pregnant woman at 36 weeks. With
permission from Dr. Robin Williams/
Science Photo Library.

Typeset by Newgen Imaging Systems Pvt Ltd.

Printed and bound in Spain by GraphyCems, Navarra

Contents

Preface

The chapters in this book appeared originally as articles in the *British Medical Journal* and were welcomed by practitioners. The articles were retuned for publication as a book, the first edition appearing in 1992. Demand asked for more and so the book was updated for a second, a third and now a fourth edition in 2002.

Antenatal care has evolved from a philanthropic service for mothers and their unborn babies to a multiphasic screening programme. Much has been added in the past few years but a lack of scientific scrutiny has meant that little has been taken away. Healthy mothers and fetuses need little high technological care but some screening is desirable to allocate them with confidence to the healthy group of pregnant women. Women and fetuses at high risk need all the scientific help available to ensure the safest environment for delivery and aftercare. The detection and successful management of women and fetuses at high risk is the science of antenatal care; the care of other mothers at lower risk is the art of the subject and probably can proceed without much technology. Midwives are practitioners of normal obstetrics and are taking over much of the care of normal or low-risk pregnancies, backed up by general practitioner obstetricians in the community and by consultant led obstetric teams in hospitals.

This book has evolved from over 40 years of practice, reading, and research. We have tried to unwind the tangled skeins of aetiology and cause and the rational from traditional management, but naturally what remains is an opinion. To broaden this, the authorship has been widened; Dr Margery Morgan, a consultant obstetrician and gynaecologist at Singleton Hospital, has joined Professor Chamberlain as a co-author, bringing with her the new skills used in antenatal care.

We thank our staff at Singleton Hospital for willingly giving good advice and contributing to this book, especially Howard Whitehead, medical photographer, and Judith Biss, ultrasonographer. Our secretaries Caron McColl and Sally Rowland diligently decoded our writings and made the script legible while the staff of BMJ Books, headed by Christina Karaviotis, turned the whole into a fine book.

Geoffrey Chamberlain
Margery Morgan
Singleton Hospital
Swansea

1 Organisation of antenatal care

Looking after pregnant women presents one of the paradoxes of modern medicine. Normal women proceeding through an uneventful pregnancy require little formal medicine. Conversely, those at high risk of damage to their own health or that of their fetus require the use of appropriate scientific technology. Accordingly, there are two classes of women, the larger group requiring support but not much intervention and the other needing the full range of diagnostic and therapeutic measures as in any other branch of medicine. To distinguish between the two is the aim of a well run antenatal service.

Antenatal clinics provide a multiphasic screening service; the earlier women are screened to identify those at high risk of specified problems the sooner appropriate diagnostic tests can be used to assess such women and their fetuses and treatment can be started. As always in medicine, diagnosis must precede treatment, for unless the women who require treatment can be identified specifically, management cannot be correctly applied.

Background

Some women attend for antenatal care because it is expected of them. They have been brought up to believe that antenatal care is the best way of looking after themselves and their unborn children. This is reinforced in all educational sources from medical textbooks to women's magazines.

Prenatal care started in Edinburgh at the turn of the 20th century, but clinics for the checking of apparently well pregnant women were rare before the first world war. During the 1920s a few midwifery departments of hospitals and interested general practitioners saw women at intervals to check their urine for protein. Some palpated the abdomen, but most pregnant women had only a medical or midwifery consultation once before labour, when they booked. Otherwise, doctors were concerned with antenatal care only "if any of the complications of pregnancy should be noticed". Obstetrics and midwifery were first aid services concerned with labour and its complications: virtually all vigilance, thought, and attention centred on delivery and its mechanical enhancement. Little attention was paid to the antenatal months.

During the 1920s a wider recognition emerged of the maternal problems of pregnancy as well as those of labour; the medical profession and the then Ministry of Health woke up to realise that events of labour had their precursors in pregnancy. Janet Campbell, one of the most farsighted and clear thinking women in medicine, started a national system of antenatal clinics with a uniform pattern of visits and procedures; her pattern of management can still be recognised today in all the clinics of the Western world.

Campbell's ideas became the clinical obstetric screening service of the 1930s. To it has been added a series of tests, often with more enthusiasm than scientific justification; over the years few investigations have been taken away, merely more added. Catalysed by the National Perinatal Epidemiological Unit in Oxford, various groups of more thoughtful obstetricians have tried to sort out which of the tests are in fact useful in predicting fetal and maternal hazards and which have a low return for effort. When this has been done a rational antenatal service may be developed, but until then we must work with a confused service that "growed like Topsy". It is a mixture of the traditional clinical laying on of hands and a

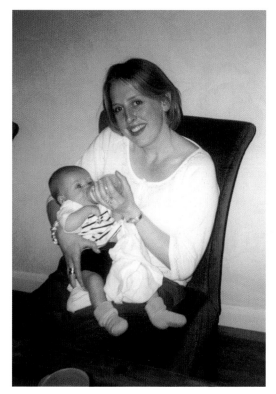

Figure 1.1 New mother and her baby

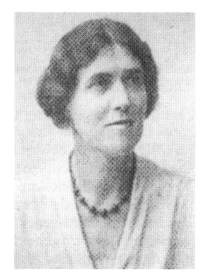

Figure 1.2 Dame Janet Campbell

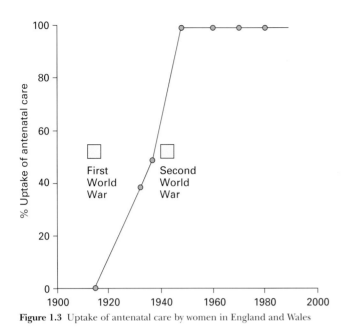

Figure 1.3 Uptake of antenatal care by women in England and Wales

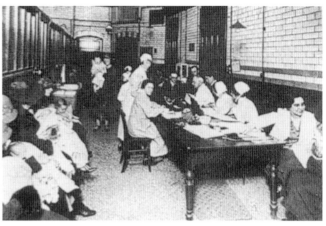

Figure 1.4 Antenatal clinics evolved from child welfare clinics, producing a prenatal version of the infant clinics

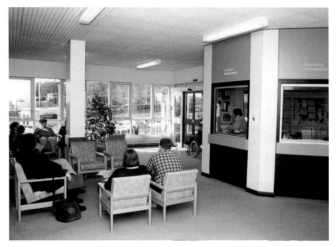

Figure 1.5 An antenatal clinic in 2001

patchily applied provision of complex tests, whose availability often depends as much on the whims of a health authority's ideas of financial priority as on the needs of the women and their fetuses.

As well as these economic considerations, doctors planning the care of women in pregnancy should consider the women's own wishes. Too often antenatal clinics in the past have been designated cattle markets; the wishes of women coming for care should be sought and paid attention to. A recurrent problem is the apparent rush of the hospital clinic. The waiting time is a source of harassment and so is the time taken to travel to the clinic. Most women want time and a rapport with the antenatal doctor or midwife to ask questions and have them answered in a fashion they can understand. It is here that the midwives come into their own for they are excellent at the care of women undergoing normal pregnancies.

In many parts of the country midwives run their own clinics in places where women would go as part of daily life. Here, midwives see a group of healthy normal women through pregnancy with one visit only to the hospital antenatal clinic.

To get the best results, women at higher risk need to be screened out at or soon after booking. They will receive intensive care at the hospital consultant's clinic and those at intermediate risk have shared care between the general practitioner and the hospital. The women at lower risk are seen by the midwives at the community clinics. Programmes of this nature now run but depend on laying down protocols for care agreed by all the obstetricians, general practitioners and midwives. Co-operation and agreement between the three groups of carers, with mutual respect and acceptance of each other's roles, are essential.

Janet Campbell started something in 1920. We should not necessarily think that the pattern she derived is fixed forever, and in the new century we may start to get it right for the current generation of women.

Styles of antenatal care

The type of antenatal care that a woman and her general practitioner plan will vary with local arrangements. The important first decision on which antenatal care depends is

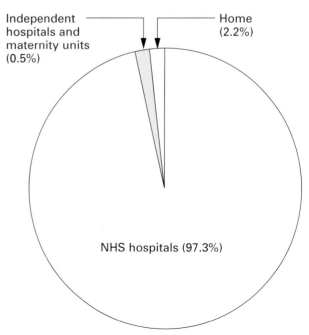

Figure 1.6 Place of birth in England and Wales, 1998

where the baby will be delivered. Ninety seven per cent of babies in the UK are now delivered in institutions, a third of the 2.2% of domiciliary deliveries are unplanned, so about 1.5% are booked as home deliveries. If the delivery is to be in an institution there is still the choice in some areas of general practitioner deliveries either at a separate unit run by general practitioners isolated from the hospital or in a combined unit with a consultant. Most deliveries take place in an NHS hospital under the care of a consultant team. A small but possibly increasing number in the next few years may be delivered in private care, by a general practitioner obstetrician, a consultant obstetrician, or an independent midwife. Recently a series of midwife led delivery units have been established with no residential medical cover.

Once the plans for delivery are decided, the pattern of antenatal visits can be worked out. If general practitioners or midwives are going to look after delivery, antenatal care might be entirely in their hands, with the use of the local obstetric unit for investigations and consultation. At the other end of the spectrum, antenatal care is in the hands of the hospital unit under a consultant obstetrician and a team of doctors and midwives, the general practitioner seeing little of the woman until she has been discharged from hospital after delivery.

Most women, however, elect for antenatal care between these two extremes. They often wish to take a bigger part in their own care. In some antenatal clinics the dipstick test for proteinuria is done by the woman herself. As well as providing some satisfaction, this reduces the load and waiting time at the formal antenatal visit.

During pregnancy there may be visits, at certain agreed stages of gestation, to the hospital antenatal clinic for crucial checks, and for the rest of the time antenatal care is performed in the general practitioner's surgery or midwives' clinic. These patterns of care keep the practitioner involved in the obstetric care of the woman and allow the woman to be seen in slightly more familiar surroundings and more swiftly. In some areas clinics outside the hospital are run by community midwives; these are becoming increasingly popular. Home antenatal care visits also take place, including the initial booking visit.

Delivery may be in the hospital by the consultant led team, by a general practitioner obstetrician, or by a midwife. It is wise, with the introduction of Crown indemnity, that all general practitioner obstetricians have honorary contracts with the hospital obstetric department that they attend to supervise or perform deliveries. About 2% of women now have a home delivery. More than half of these are planned and for this group, antenatal care may well be midwifery led (see *ABC of Labour Care*).

Box 1.1 Fees paid to GPs on the obstetrics list for maternity services April 1997

	£
Complete maternity medical services	186
Antenatal care only from before 16 weeks	100
Confinement	42
Postnatal care only	42

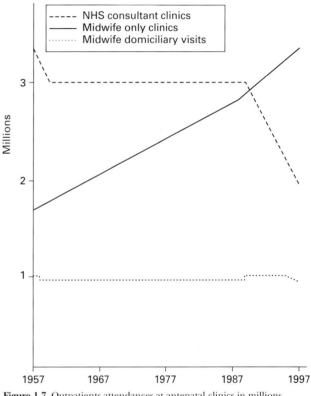

Figure 1.7 Outpatients attendances at antenatal clinics in millions, 1957–97

Early diagnosis of pregnancy

When a woman attends a practitioner thinking that she is pregnant, the most common symptoms are not always amenorrhoea followed by nausea. Many women, particularly the multiparous, have a subtle sensation that they are pregnant a lot earlier than the arrival of the more formal symptoms and signs laid down in textbooks. Traditionally, the doctor may elicit clinical features, but most now turn to a pregnancy test at the first hint of pregnancy.

Symptoms

The symptoms of early pregnancy are nausea, increased sensitivity of the breasts and nipples, increased frequency of micturition, and amenorrhoea.

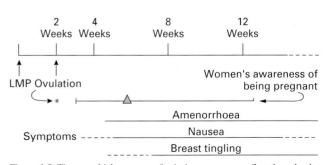
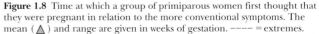

Figure 1.8 Time at which a group of primiparous women first thought that they were pregnant in relation to the more conventional symptoms. The mean (▲) and range are given in weeks of gestation. ------ = extremes.

Signs

The doctor may notice on examination a fullness of the breasts with early changes in pigmentation and Montgomery's tubercuiles in the areola. The uterus will not be felt through the abdominal wall until about 12 weeks of pregnancy. On bimanual assessment uterine enlargement is detectable before this time while cervical softening and a cystic, generally soft feeling of the uterus can be detected by eight weeks. This more subtle sign is not often sought as vaginal examination is not usually performed on a normal woman at this time.

Tests

Mostly the diagnosis of pregnancy is confirmed by tests checking for the higher concentrations of human chorionic gonadotrophin that occur in every pregnancy. The old biological tests using rabbits and frogs are now gone and have been replaced by immunological tests. These depend on the presence of human chorionic gonadotrophin in the body fluids, which is reflected in the urine. The more sensitive the test, the more likely it is to pick up the hormone at lower concentrations—that is, earlier in pregnancy.

Enzyme linked immunosorbent assay (ELISA) is the basis of many of the commercial kits currently available in chemist shops. The assay depends on the double reaction of standard phase antibody with enzyme labelled antibody, which is sensitive enough to detect very low concentrations of human chorionic gonadotrophin. Positive results may be therefore detectable as early as 10 days after fertilisation—that is, four days before the first missed period.

Vaginal ultrasound can detect a sac from five weeks and a fetal cardiac echo a week or so later (Chapter 4), but this would not be used as a screening pregnancy test.

Conclusion

At the end of the preliminary consultation women may ask questions about the pregnancy and the practitioner will deal with these. Most of these queries will be considered in the chapter on normal antenatal management. For most women the onset of pregnancy is a desired and happy event, but for a few it may not be so and practitioners, having established a diagnosis, may find that they are then asked to advise on termination of pregnancy. This they should do if their views on the subject allow; if not, they should arrange for one of their partners to discuss it with the patient. Most women, however, will be happy to be pregnant and looking forward to a successful outcome.

Recommended reading

- Cnattingius V. *Scientific basis of antenatal care.* Cambridge: Cambridge University Press, 1993.
- Cole S, McIlwaine G. The use of risk factors in predicting consequences of changing patterns of care in pregnancy. In Chamberlain G, Patel N, eds. *The future of the maternity services.* London: RCOG Press, 1994.
- Collington V. *Antenatal care.* London: South Bank University, 1998.

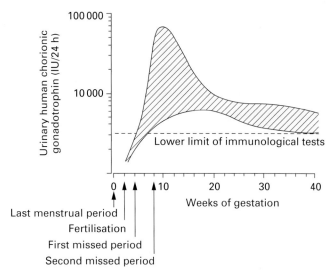

Figure 1.9 Human chorionic gonadotrophin values rise sharply in early gestation but are reduced in the second half of pregnancy. The normal range ±2 SD is shown

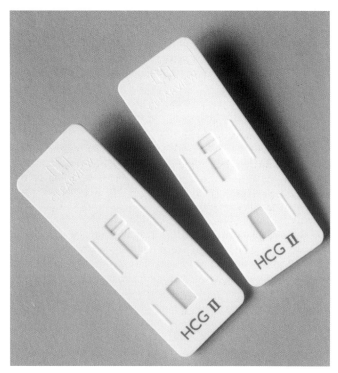

Figure 1.10 Clearview pregnancy test results. The horizontal bar in the top chamber shows that a urine sample has progressed satisfactorily from the lower chamber. A horizontal bar in the middle chamber shows a positive result (right) and its absence a negative result (left)

Antenatal care has evolved from a hospital based service to a community based service for normal women. Those with a higher risk of problems are best seen in hospital clinics.

The picture of the infant welfare clinic is reproduced by permission of William Heinemann from *University College Hospital and its Medical School: a History* by W R Merrington. The Clearview pregnancy test result is reproduced by permission of Unipath, Bedford.

2   The changing body in pregnancy

Pregnancy is a load causing alterations not just in the mother's pelvic organs but all over the body. Fetal physiology is different from that of an adult, but it interacts with the mother's systems, causing adaptation and change of function in her body. These adaptations generally move to minimise the stresses imposed and to provide the best environment for the growing fetus; they are usually interlinked smoothly so that the effects on the function of the whole organism are minimised.

Cardiovascular system

The increased load on the heart in pregnancy is due to greater needs for oxygen in the tissues.

- The fetal body and organs grow rapidly and its tissues have an even higher oxygen consumption per unit volume than the mother's.
- The hypertrophy of many maternal tissues, not just the breasts and uterus, increases oxygen requirements.
- The mother's muscular work is increased to move her increased size and that of the fetus.

Cardiac output is the product of stroke volume and heart rate. It is increased in pregnancy by a rise in pulse rate with a small increase in stroke volume. Cardiac muscle hypertrophy occurs so that the heart chambers enlarge and output increases by 40%; this occurs rapidly in the first half of pregnancy and steadies off in the second. In the second stage of labour, cardiac output is further increased, with uterine contractions increasing output by a further 30% at the height of the mother's pushing.

During pregnancy the heart is enlarged and pushed up by the growing mass under the diaphragm. The aorta is unfolded and so the heart is rotated upwards and outwards. This produces electrocardiographic and radiographic changes which, although normal for pregnancy, may be interpreted as abnormal if a cardiologist or radiologist is not told of the pregnancy.

Blood pressure may be reduced in mid-pregnancy, but pulse pressure is increased and peripheral resistance generally decreases during late pregnancy.

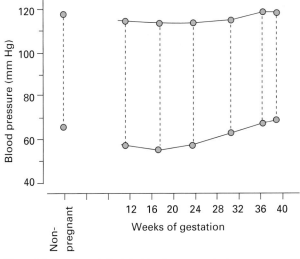

Figure 2.3 Systolic and diastolic blood pressures during pregnancy. The mid-trimester dip found in some women is seen more in the diastolic than in the systolic pressure

> Pregnancy causes physiological and psychological changes, which affect all aspects of the woman's life.

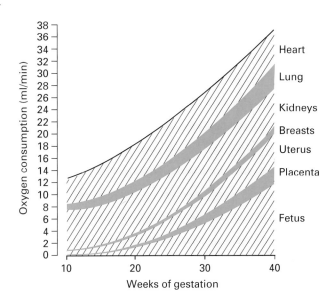

Figure 2.1 Increase in oxygen consumption during pregnancy. A major part of the increase goes to the products of conception (fetus and placenta)

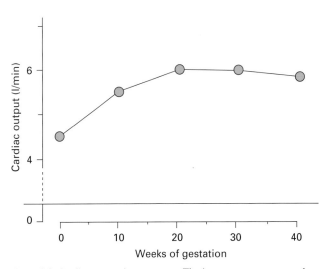

Figure 2.2 Cardiac output in pregnancy. The increase occurs very early and flattens from 20 weeks

---

Box 2.1   Changes in the ECG in normal pregnancy

- Deep Q waves in I and II
- T wave flattened or inverted in III
- ST segment depressed
- Extra-systolies frequent

Maternal blood volume increases, the changes in plasma volume being proportionally greater than the increase in red cell bulk. Hence haemodilution occurs; this used to be called a physiological anaemia, a bad phrase as it is paradoxical to have a physiological pathological process.

The heart sounds are changed.

- A systolic ejection murmur is common.
- A third cardiac sound is commonly heard accompanying ventricular filling.

The electrical activity of the heart on an electrocardiogram changes.

- The ventricles become hypertrophied, the left to a greater extent than the right and therefore left ventricular preponderance is seen in the QRS deviation.

Heart valves and chamber volumes may change during pregnancy. The heart becomes more horizontal so cardiothoracic ratio is increased and it has a straighter upper left border. These changes can be visualised by cross-sectional echocardiography, which depends on the reflection of high frequency sound from inside the heart.

Respiratory system

Box 2.2 Changes in chest radiographs in normal pregnancy

Lungs
- Show increased vascular soft tissue
- Often have a small pleural effusion especially straight after delivery

The most common changes seen on chest *x* ray films are shown in the box. Always ensure that the radiology department is told on the request form that a woman is pregnant and give an approximate stage of gestation. Only when there are strong indications should chest radiography be performed in pregnancy at all and then full radiological shielding of the abdomen must be used.

In early pregnancy women breathe more deeply but not more frequently under the influence of progesterone. Hence alveolar ventilation is increased by as much as a half above prepregnant values so that pO_2 levels rise and carbon dioxide is relatively washed out of the body.

Later the growing uterus increases intra-abdominal pressure so that the diaphragm is pushed up and the lower ribs flare out. Expiratory reserve volume is decreased but the vital capacity is maintained by a slight increase in inspiratory capacity because of an enlarged tidal volume. This may lead to a temporary sensation of breathlessness. Explanation usually reassures the woman.

Urinary system

Changes in clearance
Renal blood flow is increased during early pregnancy by 40%. The increase in glomerular filtration rate is accompanied by enhanced tubular reabsorption; plasma concentrations of urea and creatinine decrease.

The muscle of the bladder is relaxed because of increased circulating progesterone. Increased frequency of micturition due to increased urine production is a feature of early pregnancy. Later the bladder is mechanically pressed on by the

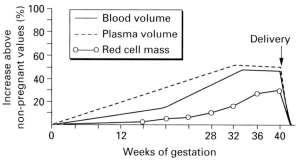

Figure 2.4 Increase in blood volume and its components in pregnancy

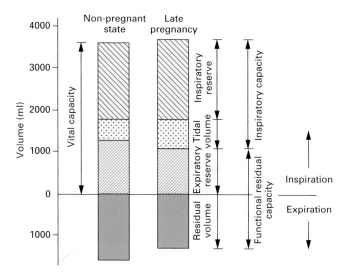

Figure 2.5 Changes in inspiratory and expiratory volumes in pregnancy

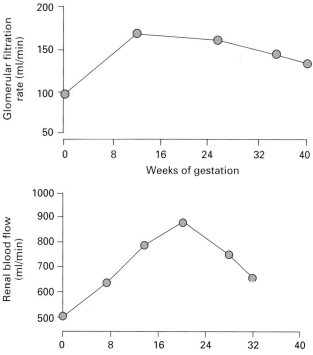

Figure 2.6 Changes in the glomerular filtration rate and in renal blood flow in pregnancy

growing uterus and the same symptoms occur but for a different reason.

The muscle walls of the ureters are relaxed by progesterone so that the ureters become larger, wider, and of lower tone. Sometimes stasis occurs in the ureters; therefore proliferation of bacteria and the development of urinary infection is more likely to occur.

Endocrine system

All the maternal endocrine organs are altered in pregnancy, largely because of the increased secretion of trophic hormones from the pituitary gland and the placenta.

Pituitary gland

The pituitary gland is increased in size during pregnancy, mostly because of changes in the anterior lobe.

Anterior lobe
- *Prolactin.* Within a few days of conception the rate of prolactin production increases. Concentrations rise until term following the direct stimulation of the lactotrophs by oestrogens. Human placental lactogen, which shows shared biological activity, exerts an inhibitory feedback effect. Prolactin affects water transfer across the placenta and therefore fetal electrolyte and water balance. It is later concerned with the production of milk, both initiating and maintaining milk secretion.
- *Gonadotrophins.* The secretions of both follicular stimulating hormone and luteinising hormone are inhibited during pregnancy.
- *Growth hormone.* The secretion of growth hormone is inhibited during pregnancy, probably by human placental lactogen. Metabolism in the acidophil cells returns to normal within a few weeks after delivery and is unaffected by lactation.
- *Adrenocorticotrophic hormone* concentration increases slightly in pregnancy despite the rise in cortisol concentrations. The normal feedback mechanism seems to be inhibited secondary to a rise in binding globulin concentrations.
- *Thyrotrophin* secretion seems to be the same as that in non-pregnant women. The main changes in thyroid activity in pregnancy come from non-pituitary influences.

Posterior lobe
There are increases in the release of hormones from the posterior pituitary gland at various times during pregnancy and lactation. These, however, are produced in the hypothalamus, carried to the pituitary gland in the portal venous system, and stored there. The most important is oxytocin, which is released in pulses from the pituitary gland during labour to stimulate uterine contractions. Its secretion may also be stimulated by stretching of the lower genital tract. Oxytocin is also released during suckling and is an important part of the let down reflex.

Thyroid gland

Pregnancy is a hyperdynamic state and so the clinical features of hyperthyroidism may sometimes be seen. The basal metabolic rate is raised and the concentrations of thyroid hormone in the blood are increased, but thyroid function is essentially normal in pregnancy.

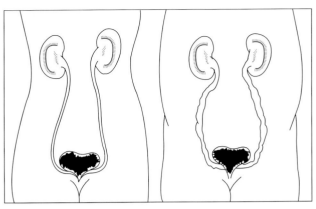

Figure 2.7 Changes in the ureters in pregnancy, during which they lengthen and become more tortuous and dilated

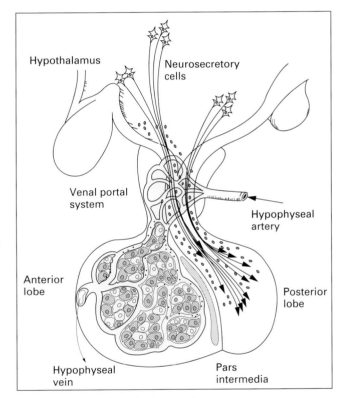

Figure 2.8 Pituitary gland showing secreting areas

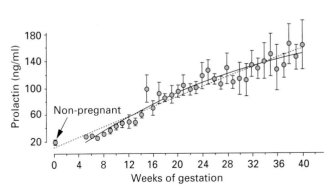

Figure 2.9 Changes in prolactin concentrations in pregnancy (means and SEMs)

In pregnancy the renal clearance of iodine is greatly increased but thyroid clearance also rises so absolute iodine levels remain in the normal range. The raised hCG levels are associated with a reduced (inside the normal range) TSH; hCG probably stimulates the gland in early pregnancy and is capable of stimulating TSH receptors.

Adrenal gland

The adrenal cortex synthesises cortisol from cholesterol. In pregnancy there is an increase in adrenocorticotrophic hormone concentration along with an increase in total plasma cortisol concentration because of raised binding globulin concentrations. The cortex also secretes an increased amount of renin, possibly because of the increased oestrogen concentrations. This enzyme produces angiotensin I, which is associated with maintaining blood pressure. Some renin also comes from the uterus and the chorion, which together produce a large increase in renin concentrations in the first 12 weeks of gestation. There is little change in deoxycorticosterone concentrations despite the swings in electrolyte balance in pregnancy.

The adrenal medulla secretes adrenaline and noradrenaline. The metabolism seems to be the same during pregnancy as before; the concentrations of both hormones rise in labour.

Placenta

The oestrogen, progesterone, and cortisol endocrine functions of the placenta are well known. In addition, many other hormones are produced with functions related to maternal adaptation to the changes of fetal growth.

In some susceptible women, progesterones may soften critical ligaments so that joints are less well protected and may separate (e.g. separation of the pubic bones at the symphysis).

Genital tract

The uterus changes in pregnancy; the increase in bulk is due mainly to hypertrophy of the myometrial cells, which do not increase much in number but grow much larger. Oestrogens stimulate growth, and the stretching caused by the growing fetus and the volume of liquor provides an added stimulus to hypertrophy.

The blood supply through the uterine and ovarian arteries is greatly increased so that at term 1.0–1.5 l of blood are perfused every minute. The placental site has a preferential blood supply, about 85% of the total uterine blood flow going to the placental bed.

The cervix, which is made mostly of connective tissue, becomes softer after the effect of oestrogen on the ground substance of connective tissue encourages an accumulation of water. The ligaments supporting the uterus are similarly stretched and thickened.

Recommended reading

- Chamberlain G, Broughton-Pipkin F, eds. *Clinical physiology in obstetrics*. 3rd edn. Oxford: Blackwell Scientific Publications, 1998.
- de Sweit M, Chamberlain G, Bennett M. *Basic science in obstetrics and gynaecology*. 3rd edn. London: Harper and Bruce, 2001.

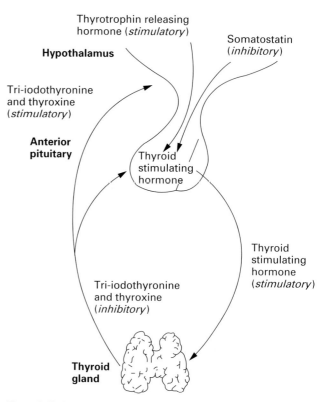

Figure 2.10 Control of thyroxine secretion in pregnancy

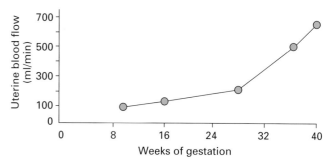

Figure 2.11 Changes in uterine blood flow in pregnancy

The wide range of normal physiological changes of gestation must be allowed for when making clinical diagnoses about diseases in pregnancy.

The figure showing the control of thyroid secretion is reproduced by permission of Blackwell Scientific Publications from *Clinical Physiology in Obstetrics* edited by F Hytten and G Chamberlain. The figure showing prolactin secretion during pregnancy is reproduced by permission of the *American Journal of Obstetrics and Gynecology* (Rigg LA, Lein A, Yen SCC, 1977;129:454–6).

3 Normal antenatal management

Antenatal care has six functions (see Box 3.1). The first two are the same as any performed in an outpatient clinic (treatment of symptoms); the second two relate to multiphasic screening, of which antenatal care was an early example; the third pair are part of health education.

> **Box 3.1 Aims of antenatal care**
> - Management of maternal symptomatic problems
> - Management of fetal symptomatic problems
> - Screening for and prevention of fetal problems
> - Screening for and prevention of maternal problems
> - Preparation of the couple for childbirth
> - Preparation of the couple for childrearing

Antenatal care in the UK is performed by a range of professionals: midwives, general practitioners, and hospital doctors. In many areas up to 90% of antenatal care is in the hands of general practitioners and community midwives. In many parts of the country midwives hold their own clinics outside the hospital or visit women at home. Probably those initially at lower risk do not need routine specialist visits for they offer little or no benefit. Many women now carry their own notes, which leads to greater understanding of what is going on.

In the UK many women book for antenatal care by 14 weeks and are seen at intervals. There is no association between the number of visits and outcome; in Switzerland there are an average of five and in The Netherlands as many as 14, but outcomes are the same. The number of visits depends on a traditional pattern laid down by Dame Janet Campbell in the 1920s (Chapter 1) rather than on being planned with thoughts relating to the contemporary scene. In an ideal world, the follow-up antenatal visits would be planned individually according to the needs of the woman and assessment of her risk.

A more rational plan of care of normal primigravidas and multigravidas is laid down in Table 3.1. With these criteria, antenatal care would be more cost effective and no less clinically useful. When pioneers have tried to reduce the number of visits from the traditional number, however, there has been resistance from older obstetricians, conventional midwives, women having babies, and their mothers, all of whom think that Campbell's by now traditional pattern must be right. A randomised controlled trial in south-east London actually found women in the fewer visits group were more likely to be dissatisfied although outcomes of the groups were the same.

As well as the clinical regimen, antenatal care now entails a whole series of special tests, but these are not generally used for the normal pregnant population.

Prepregnancy care

Some aspects of a couple's way of life may be checked before pregnancy. The man and the woman's medical and social history, and, if relevant, her obstetric career can be assessed. Immunity from infections such as rubella can be tested; alternative treatments to some longstanding conditions such as ulcerative colitis can be discussed. The possibility of a recurrence of pre-existing problems such as deep vein thrombosis can be assessed. Dietary habits and problems at work can be assessed and changes in consumption of cigarettes or alcohol may be considered. Once pregnancy has started the

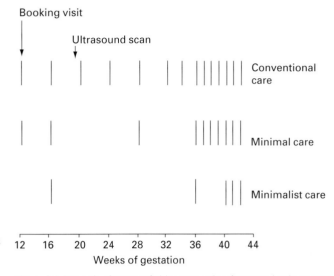

Figure 3.1 Intervals of antenatal visits: conventional pattern (top); current ideas of low risk care (middle); plan for the least number of visits (bottom)

Table 3.1 Care for normal multi- and primigravidas

Week of gestation	Main purpose of visit*
Minimum care for normal multigravidas	
12	History and examination, clarification of uncertain gestation, identification of risk factors for antenatal care and confinement, booking blood tests, booking scan in some units
	Advice on diet, drugs, work, and exercise
15–20	Downs serum screening, α Fetoprotein, anomaly ultrasound scan
22	Fundal height, baseline weight
30	Fundal height, weight gain, identification of intrauterine growth restriction and pre-eclampsia
36	Fundal height, weight gain, identification of malpresentation
40	Assessment if need for induction
Additional visits for normal primigravidas	
26	Blood pressure, urine analysis, discussion of delivery and infant feeding
34	Blood pressure, urine analysis, discussion of delivery and infant feeding
38	Blood pressure, urine analysis, discussion of delivery and infant feeding
41	Blood pressure, urine analysis, discussion of delivery and infant feeding

* Blood pressure reading and urine analysis are performed at every visit.

couple have only two options—that is, to continue or stop the pregnancy. Prepregnancy care allows more time for the correction of detectable problems and the prevention of their repetition—for example, giving supplementary folate to women whose children have abnormalities of the central nervous system. It is now recommended that extra folate is started by all women before pregnancy to avoid deficiency in very early pregnancy when the fetal neural tube is closing (21–28 days of fetal life) so as to reduce the risk of spina bifida.

Booking visit

Once pregnancy has been diagnosed, the woman usually books a visit at the antenatal clinic, the GP surgery or at home with the midwife who will lead in antenatal care. This is the longest but most important visit. It used to take place at 8–12 weeks' gestation, but in many clinics it has moved to 12–14 weeks. The woman's medical state is assessed so that the current pregnancy can be placed into the appropriate part of a risk spectrum. Baseline data are essential at this point and are obtained from the history, an examination, and relevant investigations.

History

Symptoms that have arisen in the current pregnancy before the booking visit are ascertained—for example, vaginal bleeding and low abdominal pain.

- *Menstrual history.* To assess the expected date of delivery details are needed about the last normal menstrual period including its date, the degree of certainty of that date, and whether cycles are reasonably regular around 28 days. The use of oral contraception or ovulation induction agents that might inhibit or stimulate ovulation should be discussed. A firm date for delivery from the last menstrual period can be obtained from about 80% of women.

  From this calculate the expected date of delivery with a calculator. Do not do sums in the head; this can cause trouble when a pregnancy runs over the end of a year. A woman can be told that she has an 85% chance of delivering within a week of the expected date of delivery, but we must emphasise at this point that this date is only a mathematical probability and, as with other odds, the favourite does not always win the race. Most units now rely on ultrasound to confirm gestation and alter the EDD if the scan date varies considerably, i.e. more than 10 days difference.

- *Medical history.* Specific illnesses and operations of the past should be inquired about, particularly those that entail treatment that needs to be continued in pregnancy—for example, epilepsy and diabetes.

- *Family history.* There may be conditions among first degree relatives (parents or siblings) that may be reflected in the current pregnancy, such as diabetes or twinning.

- *Sociobiological background.* Age, parity, social class, and race of the woman all affect the outcome of the pregnancy. Smoking and alcohol consumption also affect the outcome. Socioeconomic class is usually derived from the occupation of the woman or her partner. It reflects the influence of a mixed group of factors such as nutrition in early life, diseases in childhood, education, and past medical care. It also correlates with potential birth weight, congenital abnormality rates, and eventually perinatal mortality. Less strongly associated are preterm labour and problems in care of the newborn.

- *Obstetric history.* The woman's obstetric history should be discussed carefully as it contains some of the best markers for

Box 3.2 Aims of prepregnancy care

- To bring the woman to pregnancy in the best possible health
- To attend to preventable factors before pregnancy starts—for example, rubella inoculation
- To discuss diabetes and aim for excellent glycaemic control
- To assess epileptic medication in terms of fit control and teratogenicity
- To discuss antenatal diagnoses and management of abnormality
- To give advice about the effects of:
  - pre-existing disease on the pregnancy and unborn child
  - the pregnancy on pre-existing disease and its management
- To consider the effects of recurrence of events from previous pregnancies
- To discuss the use of prophylactic folate before conception

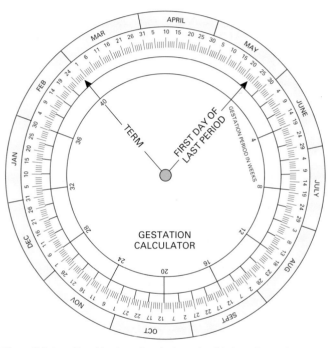

Figure 3.2 An adjustable obstetric calculator should always be used to calculate the current stage of gestation and the expected date of delivery

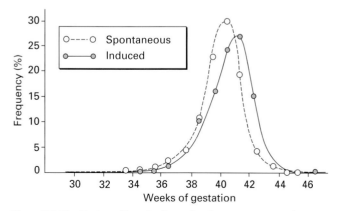

Figure 3.3 Distribution of length of gestation for spontaneous and induced single births when the last menstrual period is known (n = 16 000)

performance in the current pregnancy. If the woman has had a previous miscarriage or termination of pregnancy, the doctor should ask about the stage of gestation, and any illness afterwards. Of babies born, the progress of the pregnancy, labour, and puerperium are needed and the stage of gestation and birth weight of the infant. Intrauterine growth restriction and preterm labour may be recurrent and should be inquired about in previous pregnancies. The terms gravidity and parity are often applied to women in pregnancy. Gravidity refers to pregnancy, so anyone who is gravid is or has been pregnant. A woman who is pregnant for the first time is a primigravida. Parity refers to having given birth to a viable liveborn or a stillborn child.

Examination
A brief but relevant physical examination should be performed. The woman's height is important as it correlates loosely with pelvic size, but shoe size is a poorer predictor. Weight is less often monitored in pregnancy these days, but a booking weight will enable a Body Mass Index (BMI) to be measured. This is the weight in kilograms divided by the height squared (weight (kg)/height (cm^2)). BMI is useful in determining those at increased risk during pregnancy (over 30) who require consultant obstetric care. A value of over 39 (morbidly obese) may indicate that an anaesthetic assessment is necessary to assess potential problems in labour at delivery. The clinical presence of anaemia should be checked and a brief examination of the teeth included, if only to warn the woman to visit a dentist. Tooth and gum deterioration may be rapid in pregnancy and dental care is free at this time and for a year after delivery.

Check whether the thyroid gland is enlarged. The blood pressure is taken, preferably with the woman resting for a few minutes before. The spine should be checked for any tender areas as well as for longer term kyphosis and scoliosis, which might have affected pelvic development; the legs should be examined for oedema and varicose veins.

The abdomen is inspected for scars of previous operations—look carefully for laparoscopy scars below the umbilicus and for a Pfannenstiel incision above the pubis. Palpation is performed for masses other than the uterus—for example, fibroids and ovarian cysts. If the booking visit is before 12 weeks the uterus probably will not be felt on abdominal examination, but in a multiparous woman it may be; this should not cause the examiner to make any unnecessary comments about an enlarged uterus at this stage.

A vaginal assessment was traditionally performed at the booking visit. Its function was to confirm the soft enlargement of the uterus in pregnancy, to try to assess the stage of gestation, to exclude other pelvic masses, and to assess the bony pelvis. Many obstetricians now do not do a pelvic assessment at this stage; no woman likes having a vaginal examination and, if done in early pregnancy, it is associated in the woman's mind with any spontaneous miscarriage which may occur subsequently, even though this is irrelevant to the examination. Fetal size will soon be checked by ultrasound. Even assessment of the bony pelvis in late pregnancy may not be required as the fetal presenting part is available for check against the inlet while the effect of progesterone on the pelvic ligaments is at its maximum. By this time the woman has more confidence in the antenatal staff and is more willing to have a vaginal examination. If the head is engaged, this is a good measure of pelvis size. If it is not, a vaginal assessment may still be needed.

Table 3.2 Proportions of live births in each socioeconomic class in England and Wales adjusted by job description of husband or partner (1998)

Social class	Job description	Population having babies (%)
I + II	Professional & supervisory	25.6
IIINM	Skilled, non-manual	6.7
IIIM	Skilled, manual	16.6
IV + V	Semiskilled & unskilled	10.3
Not classifiable[*]		3.0
Not married		37.8

[*] In many surveys unemployed people are classified by their last occupation if they had one.

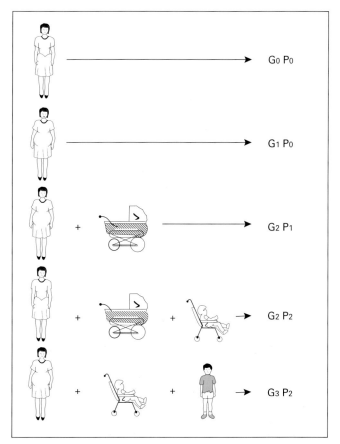

Figure 3.4 Gravidity (G) and parity (P)

Investigations

A venous blood sample is checked for:

- Haemoglobin concentration or mean cell volume (see Chapter 8).
- ABO and rhesus groups and, if relevant, rhesus antibodies. The former is to allow swifter cross-matching of blood if needed in pregnancy or labour; the latter is to warn of problems and be a baseline if a rhesus-positive fetus is in the uterus of a rhesus-negative woman.
- Antibodies to other blood groups—for example, Kell, to give warning of potential incompatibility with the fetus in the presence of less common blood groups.
- Haemoglobinopathies in women originating from Mediterranean, African, and West Indian countries.
- Syphilis. A Wassermann reaction (WR) is non-specific; most clinics now use the *Treponema pallidum* haemagglutination test to investigate more specifically, but no test can be expected to differentiate syphilis from yaws or other treponematoses.
- Rubella antibodies.
- HIV antibodies. If the woman is at risk of infection through intravenous drug misuse, having received contaminated blood transfusions, coming from parts of the world with a high HIV rate (e.g. sub-Saharan Africa), or having a partner who is HIV positive, she may request or be advised to have an HIV test. Full counselling should include her understanding the implications of both having the test and any positive result. In some parts of the UK, antenatal testing is offered to all with a modified advice service beforehand. The mother can opt out.
- Hepatitis B antibodies.
- Toxoplasmosis antibodies (if clinically appropriate).
- Cytomegalic virus antibodies (if clinically appropriate).

Later blood checks are for:

- α Fetoprotein level analysis for abnormality of the central nervous system.
- Down's syndrome serum screening by double or triple test.

The urine is checked for:

- Protein, glucose and bacteria.

Chest radiographs are rarely taken except in women from parts of the world where pulmonary tuberculosis is still endemic.

An ultrasound assessment is now performed on most pregnant women in the UK. It is best done at about

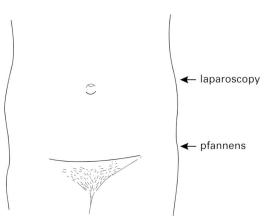

Figure 3.5 Laparoscopy and Pfannenstiel scars

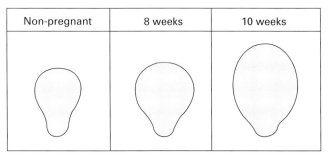
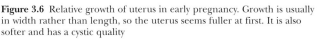

Non-pregnant	8 weeks	10 weeks

Figure 3.6 Relative growth of uterus in early pregnancy. Growth is usually in width rather than length, so the uterus seems fuller at first. It is also softer and has a cystic quality

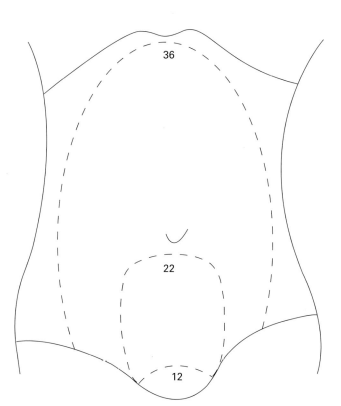

Figure 3.7 Size of uterus at various stages of gestation in pregnancy

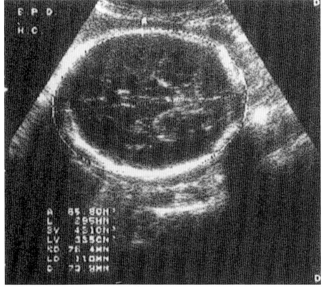

Figure 3.8 Ultrasound of fetal head showing the midline echo, the biparietal diameter of the head circumference outline

18–20 weeks to measure the biparietal diameter and so get a baseline value of fetal size and confirmation of the stage of gestation to firm up the expected date of delivery. Gross congenital abnormalities may be found (Chapter 4).

Ultrasound between 10 and 13 weeks can measure nuchal translucency, which is being evaluated as a screening test for Down's syndrome (Chapter 4). At 18 weeks congenital abnormalities such as spina bifida, omphalocele, and abnormal kidneys may be excluded. A four chamber view of the heart is also possible at this stage to exclude gross abnormalities, but details of cardiac connections may not be obvious until 22–24 weeks. Other conditions which are characterised by decreased growth such as microcephaly or some forms of dwarfism may also not be apparent until late in the second trimester.

Hence, though 16–18 weeks would be a useful time to assess gestational age by ultrasound, much later assessments are needed to assess fetal normality. In addition, more highly skilled ultrasonographers and equipment of high resolution are needed to produce scans to enable assessment of normality. Many of these ultrasound studies of fetal anatomy have been developed in specialist units with highly skilled obstetric ultrasonographers. The ordinary ultrasound service at a district general hospital cannot be expected always to provide such skill or equipment, although with increased training and better machines, some centres are now providing a fuller exclusion service at 20–24 weeks' gestation. Also at 24 weeks Doppler flow

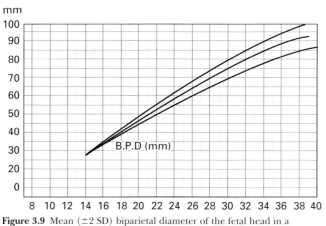

Figure 3.9 Mean (±2 SD) biparietal diameter of the fetal head in a normal population. Note the narrow range of normal values in earlier pregnancy, a great difference from that of biochemical test results

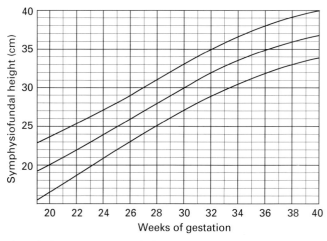

Figure 3.10 Mean (± SD) of symphysio-fundal height by weeks of gestation. Note the wide range of readings for any given week of gestation and the even wider range of expected gestation weeks for any given reading

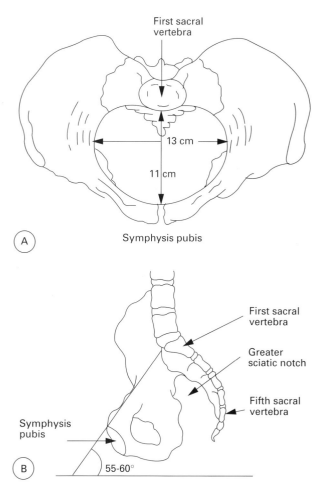

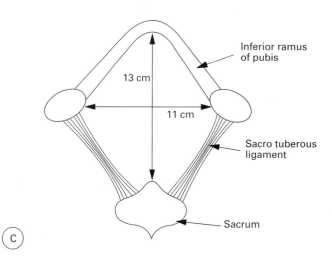

Figure 3.11 Outline of the normal bony pelvis. (A) Inlet seen from above. (B) Side view showing angle of inclination of the pelvic nm. (C) Outlet seen from below

studies may identify those mothers at risk of later hypertension or fetuses for growth restriction (Chapter 4).

Subsequent antenatal visits

At each antenatal visit an informal history is sought of events that have happened since the last attendance. The woman's blood pressure is assessed and compared with the previous readings; proteinuria and glycosuria are excluded each time. Palpation of the abdomen and measurements of the fundus above the symphysis give a clinical guide to the rate of growth of the fetus, especially if they are performed at each visit by the same observer. In later weeks the lie and presentation of the fetus is assessed. In the last weeks of pregnancy the presenting part, usually the head, is checked against the pelvic inlet to ensure that it engages. If the fetal head is not engaged by 37 weeks it is helpful to see if it will engage. To do this, the top of the couch should be propped up to 60° from the horizontal and the lower abdomen re-examined. If this small change in entry angle allows engagement of the fetal head, it will usually go down when labour contractions start. This is a simple test giving useful information about the potential of the fetal head to negotiate the mother's pelvis; it deserves wider usage in antenatal clinics.

The amount of amniotic fluid is assessed clinically and if fetal movements are seen by the observer or reported by the mother, the fetal heart need not be auscultated at the antenatal clinic. If, however, the mother reports reduced movements, the heart should be checked with a hand held Doppler fetal heart monitor and by cardiotocography so that the woman, too, can observe the heart beats and be reassured.

In a visit in the last few weeks of pregnancy a pelvic examination may be performed to check the bony pelvis, the points of importance being shown in Box 3.3. A well engaged fetal head after 36 weeks indicates, however, that the pelvis is adequate in this pregnancy and that digital assessment need not be performed. With a persistently non-engaged head or a breech presentation it should be done. Assessment of the cervix is wise at 32 weeks if the woman is at high risk of a preterm labour or is having a twin pregnancy, although it can be done in many units by vaginal ultrasound. It is also useful to assess cervical ripeness if the pregnancy is postmature after 42 weeks.

Malpositions
By 37 weeks, most fetuses will have settled into a cephalic presentation, but about 3% will still be a breech or transverse lie. Many obstetricians would offer an external cephalic version (ECV). The earlier ECV is done, the easier it is to turn the fetus but the more likely it is to turn back. Most versions are offered from 36 weeks onwards.

Before the version takes place the fetal heart is recorded for about 20 minutes and the lie checked with ultrasound. The fetal breech is then carefully disimpacted from the mother's pelvis. When above the brim, it is grasped in one hand and the head is swung round with the other hand in a series of moves so that the head is pointing downwards.

The fetal heart is checked on a cardiotocograph immediately after the version for about 20 minutes. Success rates vary between 10% and 50%.

End of pregnancy
Traditionally in Britain many obstetricians have been concerned when a singleton pregnancy goes past 42 weeks. In the 1960s the actuarial risk of perinatal mortality did sharply increase after 41 weeks, but this is no longer so and the passage

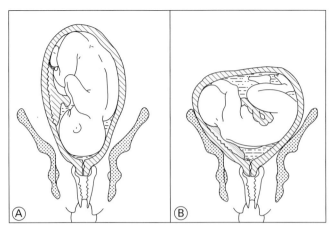

Figure 3.12 Lie of the fetus. (A) Longitudinal lie, which is deliverable vaginally. (B) Transverse lie, which if it persists has to be delivered abdominally

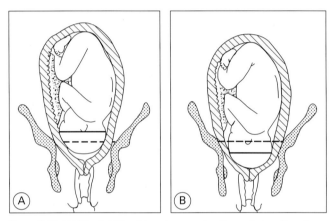

Figure 3.13 (A) The fetal head is not engaged as its maximum diameter (——) is above the inlet of the mother's pelvis (------). (B) The fetal head has descended so that its maximum diameter is below the inlet

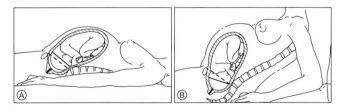

Figure 3.14 (A) The fetal head is not engaged, but when the mother sits up (B) gravity allows the head to sink below the inlet of the mother's pelvis so that the head will engage

Box 3.3 Clinical assessment of bony pelvis should include checking the:
- anteroposterior diameter from symphysis pubis to promontory of the sacrum (S1)
- curve of the sacrum
- prominence of the ischial spines
- angle of the greater sciatic notch
- width of the inferior border of the symphysis pubis
- subpubic angle

of 42 proved weeks is not used by all obstetricians as an indication for induction of labour. For example, if the cervix is not ripe some would consider it unwise to induce merely on calendar dates. Instead, the unusually long length of gestation might be used as an indication for better and more frequent fetal surveillance with Doppler and CTG rather than to take action, but this should be done at the consultant clinic in the hospital rather than in the community. The results of fetal monitoring after 42 weeks should be assessed carefully for the normal reduction of amniotic fluid volume can lead to false conclusions.

Antenatal education

Pregnancy counselling

The visits to an antenatal clinic can be a helpful time for the woman and her partner to learn about pregnancy. Formal antenatal education classes are held in most district hospitals, and couples are encouraged to attend a convenient course of counselling. Furthermore, informal discussions with midwives and doctors at the antenatal clinic are educational and much can be learnt from other mothers in the waiting time at the clinics. This is complemented by many excellent videos, which are often displayed in the antenatal waiting area.

Many good books exist about pregnancy and childbirth, offering a spectrum of styles and detail according to a woman's needs. A woman should be steered towards a well written account of what she needs in a form that best suits her lifestyle and religious observances in a language that she can understand. Plenty of such books are now available, but all hospital and obstetricians should read the material that is offered to the women who visit their clinics to make sure that they agree with and actually offer the services that the books advocate, e.g. it is no good the literature being about epidural pain relief in labour if the hospital at which the woman is booked cannot provide it.

Pregnancy social support

In the welfare state of the UK pregnant women are entitled to several social security benefits, although in many ways this country lags behind many countries in the European Union. The doctors at the clinic would do well to keep up their knowledge from time to time as benefits change rapidly according to the whims of the Department of Social Security and of their political masters. The Maternity Alliance frequently produces excellent pamphlets on these matters to help

Box 3.4 Problems with antenatal ECV

- The fetus may be too big.
- Extended legs may splint the fetus.
- The cord may be wound around the neck or limbs and so anchor the fetus.
- The abdominal muscles may be too tense to allow a grip of the fetal pole.
- Obesity may limit the grip of the fetal pole.
- The uterine muscle may contract and so resist manipulation. Try a uterine relaxant.
- Excess of amniotic fluid will allow reversion to breech presentation.
- A uterine abnormality (e.g. septum or fibroids) may not allow ECV.
- The membranes may rupture.

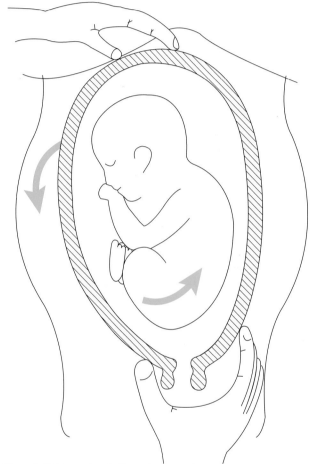

Figure 3.15 External cephalic version is usually performed by disimpacting the breech from the pelvis and then swinging the fetus through 180°

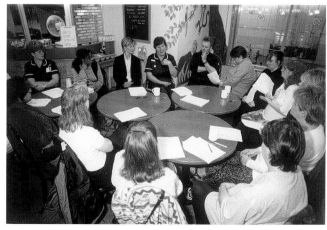

Figure 3.16 Antenatal instruction includes relaxation classes with a physiotherapist

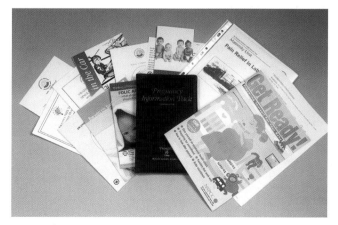

Figure 3.17 A wide variety of antenatal information books is available

15

ABC of Antenatal Care

both women and professionals keep up to date (Maternity Alliance, 45 Beech St, London EC2P 2LX).

Conclusion

The antenatal visit in the community, general practice surgery, or hospital should be friendly and held at a time when women can mix with others who are also pregnant and so informally discuss their problems. It also provides a nidus for antenatal counselling both formally at the antenatal classes and informally from staff and other women. The medical component is the core of the clinic and consists of the regular screening and assessment of symptomatic problems to bring the woman and her fetus to labour in the best state at the best time.

Antenatal care is now the cornerstone of obstetrics. Though the problems of labour are more dramatic, some of them could be avoided by effective detection and management of antenatal variations from the normal.

Recommended reading
- Fiscella K. Does prenatal care improve birth outcome? *Obstet. Gynec.* 1995;**85**:468–79.
- Hall M. Antenatal care. In Chamberlain G, ed. *Turnbull's obstetrics.* 3rd edn. London: Harper and Bruce, 2001.
- RCOG. Routine Ultrasound Screening in Pregnancy. London: RCOG, 2000.

16

4 Checking for fetal wellbeing

The great reduction in maternal mortality and morbidity in the past 30 years has allowed more attention to be concentrated on the fetus during antenatal care. Perinatal mortality has been reduced, but still in England and Wales out of 100 babies born, one will die around the time of birth, two have an abnormality, and six have a birth weight under 2500 g. With smaller family sizes in the Western world, parents expect a perfect result. General practitioners and obstetricians are performing more thorough checks to try to detect the fetuses that are likely to be at increased risk. These investigations do not replace clinical examination but provide the fine tuning of assessment. The mother still needs, however, to see someone who can talk to her and discuss the implications and results of these new tests with her.

Some groups of women are at high risk because of their medicosocial background. The extremes of maternal age (under 16 and over 35), high parity (over four pregnancies), low socioeconomic class (Office for National Statistics, social class V), and some racial groups (Pakistan-born women) seem to confer a higher actuarial risk on the babies born to such women. Consequently these women deserve extra antenatal surveillance to detect a fetus with variations from normal. Others show poor growth of the fetus in the latter days of pregnancy or develop raised blood pressure during pregnancy, two manifestations of a poor blood flow to the placental bed. Such fetuses have poor nutritional reserve—a decreased blood flow to the placental bed reduces the amounts of nutrients and oxygen. A series of tests have been developed; some of these are screening tests best applied to the total antenatal population or to a subset considered to be at higher risk. Other tests are diagnostic and specifically used for women with babies thought to be compromised clinically. All these investigations can be done in a day care unit and do not necessitate admission.

Table 4.1 Perinatal mortality in England and Wales in 1995–96 according to various maternal factors

Maternal factor	Rate per 1000 total births
Age (years)	
<20	8·5
20–24	7·1
25–29	6·6
30–34	6·7
35+	8·6
Parity	
0	6·6
1	6·4
2	8·6
≥3	15·0
Socioeconomic class	
I	5·8
II	6·0
IIIN	6·6
IIIM	7·1
IV	8·9
V	10·6
Place of mother's birth	
UK	8·2
Republic of Ireland	9·8
India	9·5
East Africa	12·4
West Indies	11·5
Pakistan	15·8

Tests in early pregnancy (up to 13 weeks)

Ultrasound
The earliest in pregnancy that the embryo may be visualised by abdominal ultrasonography is six to seven weeks; it will be shown a week earlier with a vaginal probe. At six weeks the embryonic sac can be seen but embryonic tissue cannot be confidently visualised, even with machines of high resolution and skilled ultrasonographers. By seven to eight weeks most ultrasound machines should be able to show the embryo and a fetal heart pulse can often be seen. Most obstetric departments are moving to the use of vaginal probes in early pregnancy because of the better resolution of the image. Nuchal translucency measurements are dealt with in Chapter 5.

Hormone tests
Tests are currently being developed that may be helpful in very early pregnancy to detect women who are likely to miscarry. They mostly measure proteins derived from the placenta, for example, human chorionic gonadotrophin and Schwangerschaftsprotein 1. Oestrogen and progesterone tests are too non-specific to be of prognostic value so early in gestation.

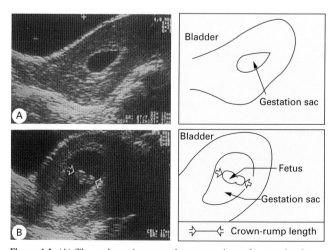

Figure 4.1 (A) The embryonic sac can be seen at six weeks gestation in decidua. As yet no fetal parts can be identified. (B) The same sac two weeks later. Fetal parts can easily be seen between the arrows. The pulsation of the fetal heart may also be seen at this time

Chorionic villus sampling
This is at present mainly used to detect chromosomal abnormalities and is considered in the next chapter.

Isoimmunisation
Maternal immune reactions may be stimulated by ante- or intrapartum fetomaternal bleeding whenever any fetal blood group factor inherited from the father is not possessed by the mother. The emphasis used to be on the Rhesus factor risk but this is rapidly being overcome by preventative anti-D gamma globulin injections given after any potential fetomaternal bleed (delivery, external cephalic version, termination of pregnancy). ABO and other blood groups become relatively more important now and antibodies for these should be screened. Management depends upon an early diagnosis of the blood groups of the mother and the presence of any antibodies. If these are detected at booking, repeat tests of antibodies should be made at intervals until the middle of pregnancy. If the antibody titre is rising the mother should be referred to a special centre capable of dealing fully with isoimmunisation.

If the rise is gradual so that the effect of the maternal antibodies passing back across the placenta is minimal to the fetus, then one might await events or stimulate an early delivery. If the position is worse, then intrauterine exchange transfusions are required. Now these are nearly always done (through a fetoscope) directly into the fetal umbilical vessels. The intraperitoneal transfusions have mostly been abandoned in the Western world. Perinatal survival rates are now reported at over 80% in even severely isoimmunised fetuses but one must remember there are complications of the invasive processes themselves. The procedure related mortality of intravascular transfusion is between 4 and 9%. The value of percutaneous transuterine umbilical artery transfusion should be compared with early delivery and performing extrauterine intravascular exchange transfusions in each centre.

Tests in mid-pregnancy (14–28 weeks)

Ultrasound
Ultrasound has become a more sophisticated tool in the past 40 years, so that by 20 weeks of pregnancy the fetus can be visualised precisely. Two separate sets of measurements are taken of the fetus to assess growth and detect malformations. The detection of malformations is the subject of the next chapter.

Growth may be determined by assessment of a series of measurements of the individual fetus at different times in pregnancy. These may then be compared with a background population to see whether the fetus is growing at the same rate as a statistically comparable group of its peers. Obviously the growth chart should relate to a population from which the fetus comes and not be taken from another population mix, although growth charts generated by ultrasonography are similar for many races except South Eastern Asians.

Crown-rump length
From 7 to 12 weeks the length of the embryo's body can be measured precisely from the crown of the head to the tip of the rump. This measurement is helpful in dating the maturity of an embryo or early fetus, but after 12 weeks it becomes less reliable because the fetus flexes and extends to a greater degree.

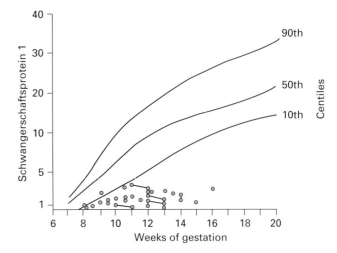

Figure 4.2 Maternal serum concentrations of Schwangerschaftsprotein 1 in pregnancies with no ultrasonic evidence of fetal heart action. This protein is made by the fetus and placenta; concentrations increase steadily through pregnancy. Many fetuses who abort spontaneously have concentrations below the 10th centile in the first weeks of gestation

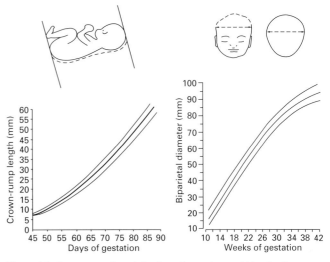

Figure 4.3 Crown-rump length by days of gestation and biparietal diameter by weeks of gestation show a narrow range inside ±2 SD of the mean, indicating a good test

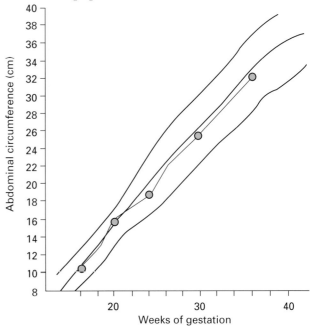

Figure 4.4 Abdominal circumference by weeks of gestation showing the mean ±2 SD. The variability is slightly wider than that in biparietal diameter but growth rates are almost linear until 38 weeks

Biparietal diameter

The distance between the two parietal eminences of the skull gives a precise measurement of fetal head size. From about 16 weeks the range of variation in a normal population widens so that in the last trimester this measurement is less useful. Early biparietal measurements are extremely helpful in dating the pregnancy with more precision even than using the date of the last menstrual period when the woman is certain of her dates. Currently, this is probably the most commonly used technique of ultrasound fetal monitoring in the Western world. If the date by ultrasound differs significantly from that expected by the last menstrual period (usually > 10 days) a revised EDD is usually calculated.

Abdominal circumference

Measurement of the fetal waist at the level of the umbilical vein provides a good assessment of the size of the fetal liver. Poor fetal nutrition prevents adequate growth of the liver following the failure to lay down glycogen. Serial measurements of abdominal circumference (or area) give good warning of placental insufficiency. A fetus who is growing well is unlikely to die except from an acute event.

Femur length

This can be readily measured from about 12 until 40 weeks. It allows a check on the somatic growth of the fetus. Impaired femur growth with skeletal dysplasia and some chromosomal anomalies invalidates this as a measure.

Amniotic fluid volume

The estimation of amniotic fluid volume is a measure of fetal metabolism. Volume is estimated by measuring the height of the largest vertical column of fluid detected by ultrasonography. A column <2 cm indicates poor production of amniotic fluid (oligohydramnios).

All these five measurements have different uses at different times of pregnancy.

Early measurements of the biparietal diameter should be used for assessing gestational age. Growth is best assessed by serial circumference measurements of the fetal head and abdomen. In late pregnancy fetal weight can be estimated by using abdominal circumference and biparietal diameter. Assessment of amniotic fluid is an attempt to study dynamic changes as it reflects fetal urine production; this is decreased in placental underperfusion.

Tests in late pregnancy (29–40 weeks)

One of the main signs of fetal wellbeing in late pregnancy is continued growth, measured by serial ultrasound examination of abdominal circumference. Readings from early pregnancy are needed to give a baseline to the growth measurements in the third trimester. This method of monitoring fetal growth has a high predictive power of detecting poor growth with high sensitivity and specificity.

Movements

Movements of the fetus are felt by the mother from about 20 weeks. In the last 10 weeks of pregnancy they may be used as

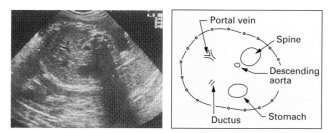

Figure 4.5 Late in pregnancy fetal growth can be detected by examining the fetal abdomen and the circumference can be marked out (by a series of dots)

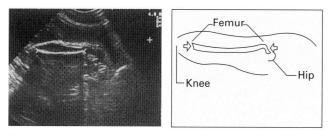

Figure 4.6 Femur length (between two arrowheads) can be measured easily by ultrasonography

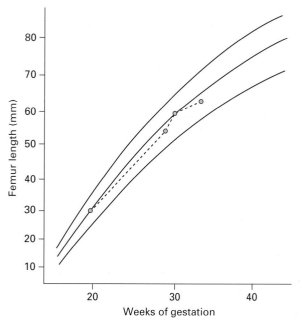

Figure 4.7 Growth in fetal femur length by weeks of pregnancy showing mean ±2 SD

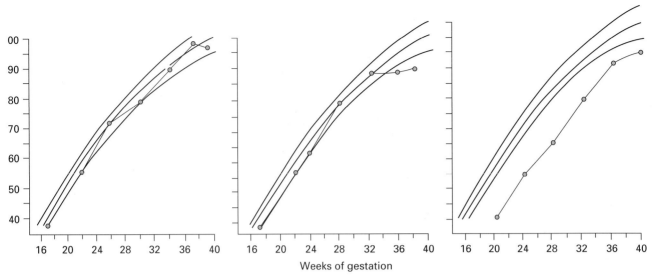

Figure 4.8 Biparietal diameter during pregnancy. Left: Growth follows the normal range of variation and stays within 2 SD of the mean. Middle: Growth tails off from about 32 weeks, the head growing hardly at all in the last weeks. Right: The first reading at 20 weeks is well outside the normal range. If the readings are put back four weeks, growth falls inside the normal range. The woman in this case was probably incorrect in her dates

a coarse measure of fetal wellbeing. Many women feel individual movements distinctly; they record these on a Cardiff Count to Ten kick chart, which estimates how long it takes for the fetus to make 10 movements. In most cases this happens within the first hour or two of the observation period, but fewer than 10 movements in 12 hours may be an early warning sign of problems. The woman should report to her obstetric department for more intensive testing, usually cardiotocography.

Cardiotocography

The fetal heart rate bears some relation to the body's response to lack of oxygen—hypoxaemia. This may be measured from 24 weeks by an external ultrasound transmitter and receiver attached to a recording system. The changes in the fetal heart rate in relation to events external to the heart rate such as uterine contractions or fetal movements can be assessed.

The baseline is important, a bradycardia being a warning sign. Episodic changes are more commonly seen, the most healthy being an acceleration; decelerations are of serious import.

Fetal heart rate varies with the balance of the sympathetic and parasympathetic nervous systems, the activity of chemoreceptors in the aorta, and concentrations of adrenaline and acetylcholine. In consequence, when the fetus is awake, baseline variability is normal. Reduced variability so that the trace becomes flat is a sign that the heart is not responding to the interaction of stimuli. This may mean accumulation of metabolic catabolites—that is, fetal acidosis. Sleep patterns need to be excluded from this diagnosis, particularly in less mature babies, as a flat trace can occur for 40 minutes or so when the fetus is asleep. The easiest way to distinguish the two is to wake the baby up by asking the mother to move around and repeat the test.

Other sinister changes include episodic decelerations with or without uterine contractions and a solitary long deceleration lasting for over five minutes.

Cardiotocograph records are widely used in the UK to monitor women at high risk in the later weeks of pregnancy to determine the best time for delivering the baby. Because of the

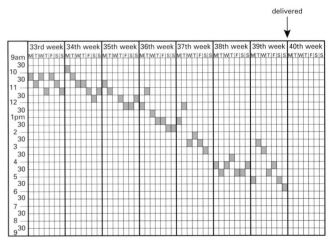

Figure 4.9 Cardiff Count to Ten kick chart. The timing of fetal movements can be graphically displayed on this chart by the mother, who is asked to contact the hospital if there are <10 movements in 12 hours

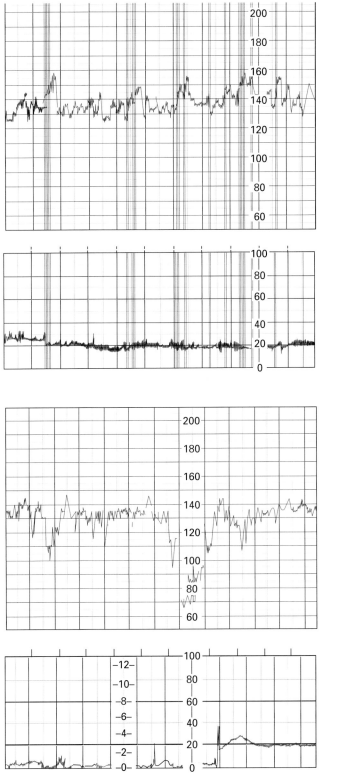

Figure 4.10 Antenatal cardiotocography showing fetal heart rate above and uterine pressure below in each trace. Top left: Fetal movements (shown by the vertical bars) are accompanied by accelerations in the heart rate. Top right: The fetus is asleep but wakes at the end of the trace. Bottom: The heart rate shows episodic decelerations, which have a bad prognosis

poor prognostic value of the individual variables that make up an antenatal cardiotocograph trace, their precise value in prediction is hard to define. A severely abnormal trace probably indicates action but an apparently normal one should not blinker decisions. The trace should be considered with other data from the pregnancy and rarely be regarded as a solitary indicant for action.

Doppler studies

The flow of blood in the arcuate branches of the uterine artery on the maternal side of the placental bed and in the umbilical artery on the fetal side can be measured by the Doppler principle.

- The afferent supply of oxygenated blood to the placental bed through the spiral arteries indicates background nutrition of the fetus in pregnancy giving longer term warning.
- The flow along the umbilical vessels indicates fetal cardiac output, a more acute measure of what is happening at the moment as reduction of flow follows poor fetal cardiac function giving more immediate warning.

Flow in other fetal vessels may help to assess the fetal state. The middle cerebral vessel, the carotid artery, the hepatic or renal vessels may be used. Ultrasound waves are beamed in and their reflected echo patterns vary with the ratio of different flows. This method of monitoring is not yet fully validated, but the interpretation of patterns is beginning to show that it is useful clinically. Abnormal waveforms from the arcuate artery are useful in predicting which women will develop severe hypertension in pregnancy. In a fetus shown to be small by ultrasound measurements, the umbilical artery waveforms help to identify the truly pathological from the constitutionally small baby. Absence or reversal of flow in the umbilical artery during diastole carries a 25–40% mortality, and up to a quarter of survivors have substantial morbidity. Conversely, small fetuses with normal umbilical waveforms have a good outcome. The middle cerebral arteries are the vessels most commonly used to assess cerebral circulation. These show a change from high to low resistance after about 30 weeks, possibly indicating dilatation as normal pregnancy progresses. During hypoxia, blood is redistributed away from the body to vital organs, achieving a brain sparing response. Measuring the ratio of flow in the middle cerebral artery to that in the aorta can give an indication of fetal hypoxia.

Invasive studies

In the second half of pregnancy fetal blood may be sampled by cordocentesis, when the oxygen saturation, carbon dioxide concentration, and concentrations of non-volatile bases such as lactate and pyruvate are measured in small blood samples. Blood is removed from the umbilical vein in the cord; the procedure carries a 1–2% risk of fetal death but the results can be invaluable about the state of fetal acid–base and blood gas concentrations. Furthermore, in some cases chromosome studies yield results that would change management.

Hormone concentrations

The estimation of oestriol concentration (or total oestrogens) in the mother's urine or blood in late pregnancy was used to give some idea of the state of the fetoplacental unit. Unfortunately, the wide variance of results within the normal range did not allow precise enough prediction and the tests have mostly been replaced by biophysical ones.

Testing for progesterone and human placental lactogen has suffered the same fate as that for oestrogen, for the same reasons.

Conclusion

The clinical assessment of the fetus can be further refined by a series of tests. Some are simple and easy to do and are used as screening tests on the whole antenatal population—for example, ultrasound for checking fetal growth. Most fetal

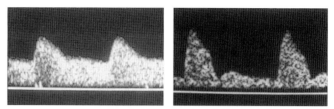

Figure 4.11 Doppler studies showing the waveforms of normal (left) and narrowed (right) arcuate arteries of the placental bed

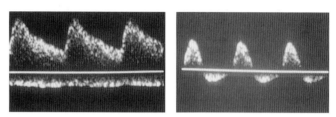

Figure 4.12 Left: Normal waveforms of the umbilical artery. Right: Severely abnormal waveforms of the umbilical artery showing reduced and even reversed flow in the diastolic phase, which suggests that the fetus is compromised

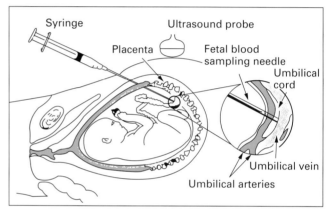

Figure 4.13 Obtaining fetal blood by cordocentesis

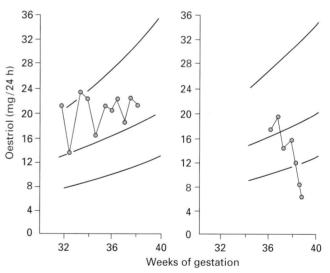

Figure 4.14 Urinary oestriol concentrations (mean (±2 SD)) during gestation. The range is much greater than that of biophysical tests. Left: Variation during a normal pregnancy. Right: Acute placental malfunction in a woman with hypertension. Currently, signs of fetal compromise measured biophysically would have indicated that she be delivered before the last oestriol readings were available

Fetal investigations should be considered to be either screening, for use in large populations, or specifically diagnostic, for use in a selected number of fetuses in which there is clinical suspicion of significant pathological lesions.

investigations, however, should be kept for women who are at high risk of specific conditions—for example, doppler studies in a fetus thought to be small.

The development of more complex biophysical tests has led to a concentration of antenatal care for women at high risk in specialist hospital units. Many district general hospitals do not have all the facilities required so the proper use of regional centres for specialist tests must be encouraged. It may be unpleasant for a woman to have to move from her home area to a centre 40 or 60 km away, but this is usually acceptable if benefits of fetal diagnosis and treatment can be explained by the doctor or midwife so that the woman realises she is helping her baby. Unfortunately, resources and skills cannot be spread uniformly throughout the country. A natural resistance to the new does happen in medicine, but it is Luddite to ignore new investigations merely because they were developed after the practitioner qualified.

Recommended reading

- Gaziano E. Antenatal ultrasound of fetal Doppler. *Clin Perinatal* 1995;**22**:111–40.
- Ingemarsson I, Ingemarsson E, Spencer J. *Fetal heart rate monitoring*. Oxford: Oxford Medical Publications, 1993.
- RCOG. *Use of anti D immunoglobin for Rh prophylaxis*. Guidelines no. 22. London: RCOG, 1999.

5 Detection and management of congenital abnormalities

A congenital abnormality in their expected baby is greatly feared by couples; we are not many generations away from the superstitious who looked on malformation as a retribution for moral misbehaviour. Congenital abnormalities are still one of the major causes of perinatal mortality and morbidity.

The known causes of abnormality are genetic or environmental. Genetic abnormality depends on the chromosomes we inherit from our parents together with the breaks and realignments occurring at fertilisation. As well as the single gene diseases and those following chromosomal rearrangement at meiosis, a large number of conditions appearing in later life, such as hypertension and some cancers, are genetically associated. A whole new philosophy of preventive care is opening. Maternal ageing also increases the risk of abnormalities in genes. A good account of genetic abnormalities is found in the *ABC of Clinical Genetics*.

If parents ask about the risks of recurrence of congenital abnormality, having already had one child with a problem, there are two sets of variables the practitioner has to consider: those who may have a similar defect and those who may have a different defect. Whilst the former are fairly high there is also a small increased risk of new defects.[1]

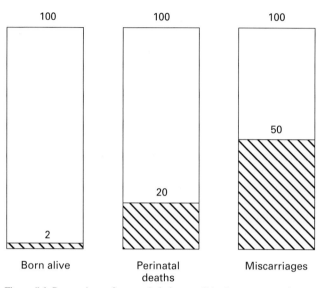

Figure 5.1 Proportions of congenital abnormalities by outcomes of pregnancy

Table 5.1 Risks of similar and dissimilar congenital abnormalities in the second infants of mothers with an affected first infant*

Defect in first infant	Defect in second infant	
	Similar defect relative risk†	Dissimilar defect relative risk†
Talipes	7·3 (5·9–9.1)	1.4 (1.0–1.7)
Limb defect	11.3 (7.2–17.0)	2.4 (1.7–3.3)
Cardiac defect	6.0 (2.2–13.0)	1.1 (0.5–1.9)
Cleft lip	31.4 (19.0–52.0)	2.2 (0.6–2.2)
Cleft palate	44.5 (9.0–13.4)	0.7 (0.1–2.5)

* Based on 1.5 million births in Norwegian Medical Birth Registry.[1]
† 95% confidence intervals for the odds ratios in parentheses.

Environmental factors interfere with embryonic development at a precise stage of organogenesis. They are difficult to pinpoint and often are misassociated. Obvious insults such as exposure to thalidomide, x rays, and rubella can be identified; more difficult is the precise place of factors such as organic solvents in the cleaning industry and infections such as toxoplasmosis, cytomegalovirus, and parvovirus.

An antenatal service should aim at diagnosing congenital abnormalities as early as possible. Though the ideal treatment is prevention, this is too late by the time the woman joins the antenatal clinic. If an abnormality can be detected early the couple may be offered the choice of a termination of pregnancy. This is allowed in the UK under statutory grounds of the modified Abortion Act 1967 with no gestational age limit (Fig. 5.3).

Not all couples want to abort their unborn child even if it has an abnormality. Antenatal diagnostic facilities should be made available not only to those who wish a termination pregnancy if an abnormality is found but to affected couples for the reasons given in Box 5.1.

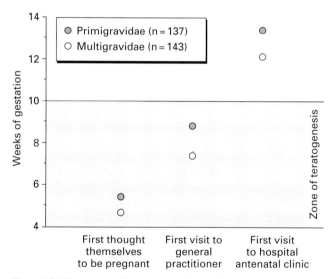

Figure 5.2 When women joined antenatal care. By the time they arrived in the hospital clinic it was far too late for advice to have any influence on the embryo in the first trimester. Maybe the GP visit is the time to provide help

Box 5.1 Reasons for providing an antenatal diagnosis of congenital defect to all relevant couples

- It gives the couple more time to accustom themselves and other children in the family to the idea that an abnormal child is to be born.
- If the abnormality is not lethal, early diagnosis allows plans to be made for delivery in a centre where full treatment may be given early.
- If the abnormality is serious and possibly lethal, counselling for termination of pregnancy can be considered.
- If one of a pair of twins shows a serious anomaly, the option of fetocide can be discussed.

Currently antenatal screening for congenital abnormalities is still mostly concerned with detection of malformations of the central nervous system, the skeleton, and abnormalities of chromosomal origin. The diagnosis of abnormalities of the cardiovascular, alimentary, and urinary tracts is improving; many of these abnormalities are now treatable by neonatologists and paediatric surgeons. Hence, if diagnosed in pregnancy, a woman can be transferred to a hospital where such skills are found. She can have antenatal counselling and the baby can be treated at the best time after the delivery, promptly if necessary.

Testing in early pregnancy

Chromosomal problems

To examine fetal chromosomes, fetal cells are required. In chorionic villus sampling (CVS) a minute piece of trophoblast tissue is removed for examination of the chromosomes in the cell nucleus and, with increasing confidence, DNA assessment. Such sampling is commonly performed at 10–12 weeks of gestation, and a preliminary result is available a couple of days after the test compared with the delay of at least 14 days for amniocentesis. Sampling is under ultrasound control by the transcervical or the transabdominal route (Fig. 5.4). Reports of fetal damage being associated with the transabdominal approach before 10 weeks gestation have led to reservations about its use.[2] There has been a concomitant trend to use amniocentesis at an earlier stage. It is now possible to get a good sample of cells from amniotic fluid safely at 12–13 weeks, so this too is swaying some against CVS.

The attraction of CVS and its quicker results are offset by the higher risks of stimulating a miscarriage. Abortion rates associated with CVS are 2–4% compared with 0.3–1.0% with 16 week amniocentesis. At 10–12 weeks of gestation, however, the rate of spontaneous miscarriage is biologically much higher than at 16 weeks, so the comparison is not only of techniques. Many obstetric units are now using CVS for women at high risk, and with experience the miscarriage rates would be expected to fall.

A nationally organised randomised controlled trial found that CVS had more problems than amniocentesis in diagnostic accuracy, safety, and the need for further testing. However, the obvious advantages of earlier testing and receiving a quicker answer must be weighed against this. Doctors would do well to refer women asking for either procedure to a department of obstetrics that performs both and will give impartial and balanced advice in each individual case. In many centres both tests show similar risk rates.

Trisomy 21 (Down's syndrome) is much commoner in women over 35, but still half of the babies with this condition are born to women under that age. Although the risks to mothers under 35 are less, the overall number of babies born is much greater. To negate this, simple screening is required since both CVS and amniocentesis are unsuitable, invasive procedures

We hereby certify that we are of the opinion, formed in good faith, that in the case

of ....
(Full name of pregnant woman in block capitals)

of ....

....
(Usual place of residence of pregnant woman in block capitals)

(Ring appropriate letter(s))

A the continuance of the pregnancy would involve risk to the life of the pregnant woman greater than if the pregnancy were terminated;

B the termination is necessary to prevent grave permanent injury to the physical or mental health of the pregnant woman;

C the pregnancy has NOT exceeded its 24th week and that the continuance of the pregnancy would involve risk, greater than if the pregnancy were terminated, of injury to the physical or mental health of the pregnant woman;

D the pregnancy has NOT exceeded its 24th week and that the continuance of the pregnancy would involve risk, greater than if the pregnancy were terminated, of injury to the physical or mental health of any existing child(ren) of the family of the pregnant woman;

E there is a substantial risk that if the child were born it would suffer from such physical or mental abnormalities as to be seriously handicapped.

Figure 5.3 Part of the modified certificate A of the Abortion Act 1967 (revised 1991)

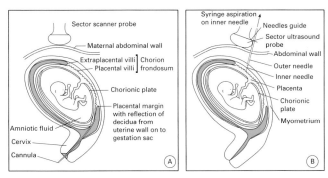

Figure 5.4 Chorionic villus biopsy. Under ultrasound guidance there can be (A) a transcervical approach of the cannula to the edge of the developing placenta or (B) a transabdominal aspiration by needle from the middle of the trophoblast mass

Table 5.2 Refining the risk of Down's syndrome by comparing age alone with results of age and the Triple Test using levels (multiples of mean, MoM) of α fetoprotein (α FP), oestriol, and human gonadotrophin (hCG)

Age alone			Age (years)				
			≤20	21–25	26–30	31–39	≥40
			1:1530	1:1350	1:900	1:385	1:110
Age and triple test (MOM)							
α FP	Oestriol	hCG					
>0.5	>0.5	<2.0	1:1200	1:100	1:70	1:30	1:10
>2.0	>2.0	<0.5	1:140 000	1:120 000	1:84 000	1:35 000	1:1000

that are very labour intensive. Hence the combination of biochemical tests of maternal blood in early pregnancy to screen for Down's syndrome is widely used. Maternal α fetoprotein, human chorionic gonadotrophin, and oestriol concentrations are measured and the relative risks of each are computed along with the risk advanced by the mother's age at any given gestation. A double test leaves out the oestriol estimation. A combination of risk values for these four markers plus age gives a detection rate (see Table 5.2) and provides the odds of the fetus being affected with Down's syndrome given a procedure screening result. Thus women can be identified who are at high enough risk to justify the hazards and costs of amniocentesis or CVS, the only currently practical ways of getting fetal cells and performing a diagnostic procedure. If the gestational dates used are derived from ultrasound rather than clinical measures, a 10% increase in detection rate is found. Current research is assessing additional markers in both urine and blood at 12 and 15–16 weeks gestation, including pregnancy associated protein A, inhibin A, and urinary β hCG.

Such screening should be offered in all women irrespective of age. It is illogical to restrict it to the over 35-year-olds. As a screening method, maternal age and biochemical estimates would replace the poorer age-only based screen, giving the woman a more precise prognosis of risk and so allowing a more informed decision before going into the diagnostic test of checking fetal chromosomes.

Fetal cells can be detected in the mother's serum as early as 6 week gestation. Though few, they can be identified and isolated. With DNA reduplication, the chromosomal material can be increased and examined. So far male cells have been identified; only female adult cells are present in the mother, any with male chromosomes must have crossed the placenta from the male fetus. Soon DNA manipulation could allow chromosomal abnormalities to be detected and may remove the need for amniocentesis but this is not yet clinical practice.

Ultrasound tests

The association of ultrasound measured fetal nuchal translucency with Down's syndrome (Table 5.3) and other chromosomal abnormalities has a sensitivity exceeding that of serum screening and a high predictive value. Equally importantly, nuchal translucency measurements correlate with serum screening levels, so that the combination of both tests might increase sensitivity and specitivity.

The big advantage is that this is a non-invasive test done at about 10 weeks of gestation so might be used as a screening test to indicate which women should go forward for fuller chromosome analysis by CVS or amniocentesis.[3, 4] However, sensitivity varies widely according to the skill of the ultrasonographers and the equipment they use.

Those experienced in using the test claim that sensitivity will improve and are now adding a series of other ultrasound markers of Down's syndrome (Box 5.2) in later pregnancy.

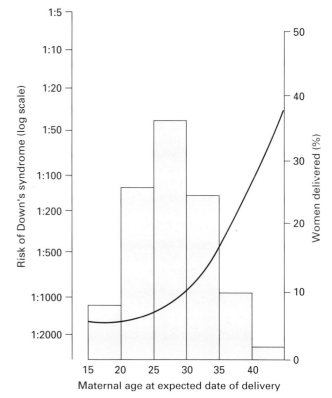

Figure 5.5 Risks of Down's syndrome. The risk increases after 35 and sharply after 40. The percentage of women in the UK who deliver by each age group is also shown. Although the risk is high after 40, the numbers of women delivering are small

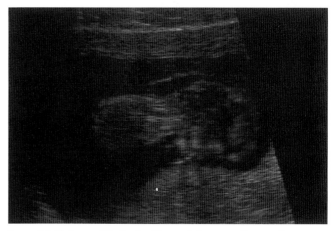

Figure 5.6 Oedema of the back of the neck shows on ultrasound; increased oedema is associated with increased rates of chromosomal abnormalities

Table 5.3 Rising risk of Down's syndrome with increase in nuchal skin fold oedema (from Nicholaides *et al. Br J Obs & Gyn* 1995;101:782–786)

Nuchal oedema (mm)	Relative risk of Trisomy 21
<3	0.2
3	3.2
4	19.8
5	28.6
>5	45.2

Box 5.2 Ultrasound soft markers of Down's syndrome
- Dilated renal pelves
- Nuchal translucency/thickness
- Choroid plexus cysts
- Echogenic bowel
- Short femur

Testing in mid-pregnancy

Structural abnormalities

Open neural tube defects such as anencephaly and open spina bifida allow α fetoprotein to escape from cerebro-spinal fluid into the amniotic fluid, whence it is absorbed into the maternal blood, producing higher than normal concentrations. This is the basis of serum α fetoprotein screening performed between 14 and 16 weeks. It is virtually non-invasive, entailing only a blood sample, and has a high predictive value. Fetal gestational age must be estimated by ultrasonography. False positive results can be caused by multiple pregnancy, a dead fetus, bleeding behind the placenta (which may manifest as a threatened miscarriage), and a few rather rarer abnormalities of the fetus such as gastroschisis.

If the serum α fetoprotein concentration is high a special ultrasound scan may be performed to examine the spine and head carefully at 16–17 weeks of gestation. In some units ultrasound alone is used for the detection of neural tube defects.

By 20 weeks the fetus can be seen clearly on ultrasonography and many neural tube defects will have been detected. At this gestation the heart can be examined and the four chambers identified. The appearance and orientation of

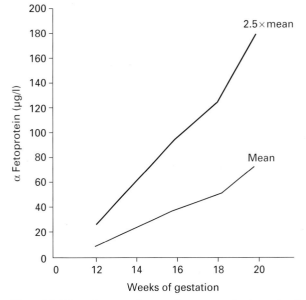

Figure 5.7 Maternal serum α fetoprotein concentration by weeks of gestation. The lower line is taken as the upper boundary of the normal group so it is important to date the pregnancy precisely – that is, by ultrasound measurement of the biparietal diameter. This is magnified by ×2.5 the mean to exaggerate differences

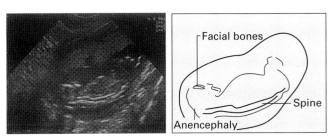

Figure 5.8 Ultrasound scan of a fetus with a sacral meningocele taken at 19 weeks

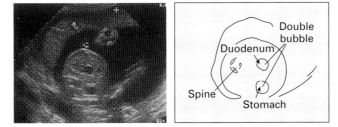

Figure 5.11 Ultrasound scan showing male genitalia resting on the section of the thigh in a fetus of 30 weeks

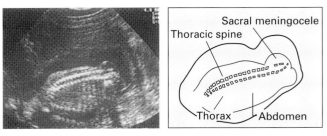

Figure 5.9 Scan of a fetus with anencephaly taken at 17 weeks

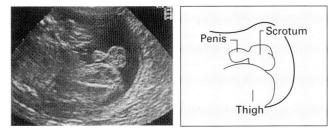

Figure 5.12 Double bubble effect of duodenal atresia, with the lower bubble in the stomach and the upper bubble in the duodenum. Normally continuity can be traced between these two bubbles

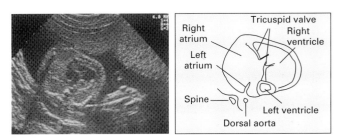

Figure 5.10 Ultrasound scan of the heart of a fetus with mitral atresia taken at 23 weeks gestation

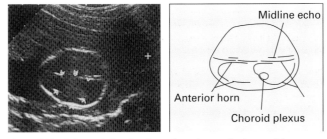

Figure 5.13 Hydrocephalus showing enlarged posterior horn of the ventricle (between single arrows) and anterior horn (between double arrows)

the great vessels can also be checked so that major cardiac abnormalities can be excluded. Limbs can be seen to exclude any shortening and, if relevant, the sex of the child may be determined by sighting the external genitalia.

Later still the kidneys may be assessed for cysts or damming back of urine, producing hydronephrosis. Blockage in the intestinal tract can be checked by the presence of bubbles of fluid in the stomach, duodenal, or large bowel area. The cerebral cortex and ventricles can also be easily visualised and measured; any persistent choroid plexus cysts can be detected. Structural abnormalities of the limbs and digits will be apparent later and some degrees of cleft lip or palate can be found.

The volume of amniotic fluid can be calculated from measurements inside the uterine cavity or more pragmatically by measuring the longest column at the maximum diameter of the largest fluid pool.

These investigations permit a thorough knowledge of the unborn child. Many of the skills are available in the ultrasound departments of district general hospitals, but there is more expert back up at the special obstetric ultrasound clinics of tertiary referral hospitals.

Chromosomal abnormalities

In mid-pregnancy the chromosomal state of the fetus may be checked from cells removed at amniocentesis. Early amniocentesis (before 14 weeks) appears to be associated with significant problems including increased fetal loss, fetal talipes, and difficulty with culturing the chromosomes. New polymer chain reaction techniques have enabled preliminary results to be available within 24 hours but the full results for chromosome cultures still take some weeks.

The commonest use of amniocentesis is for the diagnosis of Down's syndrome (trisomy 21), and in most parts of England and Wales women over the age of 35 are offered this screening test. Serum screening of hCG, α fetoprotein and oestriol is used to determine those at higher risk of Down's syndrome. Amniocentesis is an invasive procedure with a small risk of spontaneous miscarriage (0.3–1.0% above background rate of miscarriage). This risk is less if the procedure is done under ultrasound guidance by an experienced obstetrician (0.3–0.8%).

Occasionally from about 20 weeks of pregnancy it is necessary to be certain that the fetus has normal chromosomes if a high risk pregnancy is to be continued under adverse circumstances. It is wise to know that the baby is normal before putting the mother through many weeks of anxiety and possibly a caesarean section. The white cells of fetal blood can be obtained at cordocentesis by penetrating the umbilical cord where the vessels are held firmest, close to the placenta or to the fetal belly wall. Chromosome examination of the white blood cells gives a result fairly speedily (two or four days).

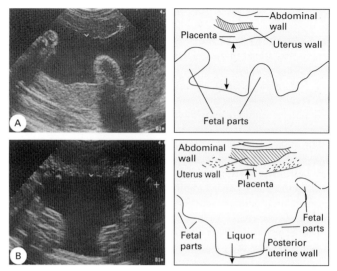

Figure 5.14 Amniotic fluid estimation. (A) The largest pool has the longest column of 5.3 cm (between the arrows); this is normal. (B) In polyhydramnios the longest pool between the arrows has a column of 9.1 cm. Generally 8.0 cm is taken as the upper limit of normal

(NORMAL ✓ NOT SEEN *NS*)

DATE .... GESTATIONAL AGE BY EDD .... wks			
CRANIUM		HEART – 4 chambers	
VENTRICLES		STOMACH	
CEREBELLUM		KIDNEYS	
SPINE		BLADDER	
4 LIMBS SEEN		CORD INSERTION	

Figure 5.15 A typical anomaly checklist to be completed at the 18–22 week ultrasound scan

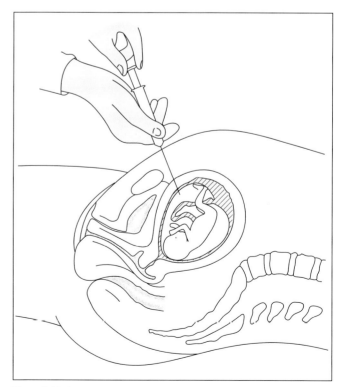

Figure 5.16 Amniocentesis under local anaesthesia. The fluid withdrawn (about 10–15 ml) is spun down and the cells are used for culture

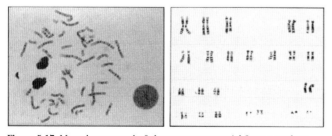

Figure 5.17 Metaphase spread of chromosome material from a nucleus after culture. The chromosomes are photographed and the print cut out and arranged in pairs to show the normal arrangement for a female, two X chromosomes at the end of the bottom grouping

Abnormalities of the central nervous system
The total number of abnormalities of the central nervous system in England and Wales has fallen since the early 1970s. Data are based on three sources:

- notification of termination of pregnancy for abnormalities of the central nervous system;
- death certification of stillbirths and neonatal deaths because of abnormalities;
- notification of abnormalities of babies who live.

Whilst rates are at 1.75 per 1000 in Wales, there is a differential in the south of Britain, where the proportional decrease is even greater. In many parts of southern England, the rate of abnormalities of the central nervous system is less than 1 per 1000. At this level a screening programme that used α fetoprotein might do more harm than good because action might be taken on false positive results. Many authorities have abandoned biochemical screening for these reasons.

Ultrasound as a screening test for anencephaly has good results, and when modern, high resolution equipment is available spina bifida can be detected. Although the special skills and equipment are currently not always available in DGH ultrasound clinics, regional centres do provide them.

Availability of tests

Biochemical screening for abnormalities of the central nervous system and for Down's syndrome is patchy and varies from one district health authority to another. The reasons lie not just in the whims of economic diktat but with variations in the interpretation of epidemiological data.

Congenital abnormalities

Down's syndrome
As explained previously, the risks of Down's syndrome are greater in women over 35, but because most babies are born to women under this age about half of the babies with the syndrome will be missed if age is used as an indicator for fetal chromosome tests. The use of serum screening with ultrasound has offered younger women the option of testing for Down's syndrome, although costs will have to be considered. To detect one affected fetus it now costs about £15 000 to screen for Down's syndrome. Some health authorities would set this against the cost of maintaining a child born with Down's syndrome for the rest of his or her life in an institution, probably between £17 000 and £30 000. The cost of diagnosis, however, comes from one year's budget, whereas the cost of maintenance is spread over many years' budgets in the future; local health authorities are forced into this philosophical financial juggling.

Many units in the UK have introduced serum screening enabling those women considered to be at high risk by age alone to be reallotted to a lower risk group if the results are favourable. With recent advances in early ultrasound, it is likely that a combination of serum screening and measurement of the nuchal fold will produce the best pick-up rate for the lowest level of false positives.

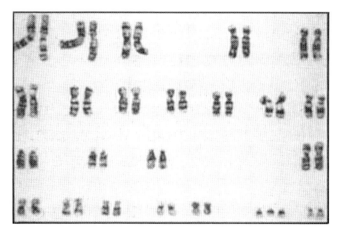

Figure 5.18 Chromosomes of a woman with trisomy 21. The last but one grouping (position 21) has three chromosomes instead of two

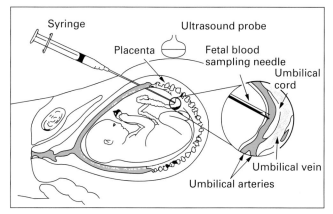

Figure 5.19 Cordocentesis

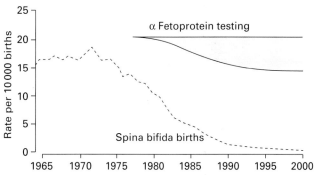

Figure 5.20 Birth prevalence of spina bifida in England and Wales. A slight reduction has occurred from the mid-1960s, becoming sharper from 1973. Testing for α fetoprotein, although described in the early 1970s, was not widespread until the 1980s and so there may be a coincident factor in this reduction as well as the effect on screening. Many think this is due to an improved diet for the women of this country

Conclusion

At first the antenatal detection of congenital abnormalities may seem to lead only to a nihilistic outcome, but the diagnosis can lead to other lines of management such as the preparation for early paediatric surgery or, in future, to genetic engineering. This is unlikely to be of any help once the embryo has started its development, but work done now on forming embryos can be extrapolated back to research on the oocyte. Here recombinant DNA technology may be used to change the affected part of a chromosome before cell development starts, thus producing a normal fetus. Such technology obviously needs to be controlled by society to help couples who previously had no chance of producing a normal baby.

> **Detection of fetal abnormalities in early pregnancy need not just lead to termination of pregnancy. Many results confirm normality and so reassure the mother. Even when positive, the results lead to the provision of better neonatal services when the affected baby is born.**

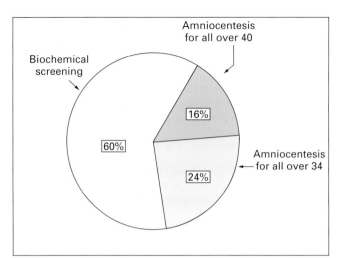

Figure 5.21 Detection rates of Down's syndrome comparing age as the only criterion with the results of triple biochemistry screening to indicate amniocentesis

References

1 Lie R, Wilcox A, Skjaerven R. Population based study on the risks of recurrent birth defects. *New Engl J Med* 1994;**331**:1–4.
2 Firth HV, Boyd TA, Chamberlain P, Mackenzie IZ, Linderbaum RH, Huson SM. Severe limb abnormalities after chorion villus sampling at 56–66 days' gestation. *Lancet* 1991;**337**:762–3.
3 Brizot M, Snijdes R, Butler J, *et al.* Maternal serum hCG and fetal nuchal translucency thickness for prediction of fetal trisomies in the first trimester of pregnancy. *Br J Obstet Gynaec* 1995;**102**:127–32.
4 Bewley S, Robers I, MacKinson A, Rodeck C. The use of first trimester measurements of fetal nuchal translucency. Problems of screening a general population. *Br J Obstet Gynaec* 1995;**102**:386–8.

Recommended reading

- Grundzinskas J, Ward R. *Screening for Down's syndrome in the first trimester.* London: RCOG Press, 1997.
- Hill L. Detection neural tube defects. In Rodeck C, Whittle M, eds. *Fetal medicine.* London: Harcourt Brace, 1999.
- Ott W. *Clinical obstetrical ultrasound.* Bristol: Willey, 1999.
- RCOG. *Amniocentesis.* Guidelines no. 8. London: RCOG, 1996.
- RCOG Working Party. *Ultrasound screening for fetal abnormalities.* London: RCOG, 1997.

6   Work in pregnancy

Both the proportions and numbers of women in the paid workforce have been increasing in England and Wales since before the second world war. In 2000 46% of the workforce were women, many in part-time posts, and this statistic has important implications for childbearing and reproduction.

Other important changes are women working longer in pregnancy and the postponement of starting a family to an older age. Three-quarters of couples need two incomes to pay the mortgage and other loans. When the woman becomes pregnant she receives maternity benefits, but these are poor compared with those in other European countries and income will be reduced. Every woman is entitled to 18 weeks of maternity leave. During the first six weeks of this she gets 90% of her average pay and for the next 12 weeks she gets standard maternity pay which is currently £62.20, going up to £75 per week in 2002 and £100 in 2003, hence the total standard maternity pay is for 18 weeks for those who have worked before pregnancy. Maternity allowance is separate and may be claimed. Currently this is £62.20 a week for women who are employed in pregnancy. There are no deductions for tax or National Insurance contributions. This is paid for 18 weeks when the woman is not working.

These and other allowances change often and practitioners would be wise to update themselves from time to time. Details can be obtained from the local Social Security Office or Factsheets from the Maternity Alliance (45 Beech Street, London EC2P 2LX) who provide up-to-date information on this and many other matters. They are most helpful to the cause of women who work in pregnancy.

In the UK the number of women over the age of 35 having babies has increased in the past 30 years because the years of reproduction are those of career advancement and each pregnancy becomes a gap in climbing the ladder of promotion.

Two-thirds of the women in the paid workforce currently continue to work longer into pregnancy than women did in the 1960s. Whereas some stop around the 28th week of pregnancy, most of them continue into the 34th or 35th week. Women are entitled to maternity leave for six weeks on 90% and 12 weeks on £62.20. This can start from 11 weeks before the expected time of delivery, as certified by a doctor or midwife on the MATB1 form. Most women, however, prefer to have as much time as possible with their newborn child after delivery and so do not leave work early.

In certain circumstances a woman leaving her job during pregnancy is entitled to return after maternity leave up to one year after delivery. The employer must, however, employ more than five people and the woman must have worked with the employer for two years in a full-time job or longer in a part-time post. If she wishes to protect her job she must give her employer 21 days' notice of her intent to stop working and she cannot leave until the 28th week of pregnancy. In return for this the employer must keep the job open for a year and, though the exact job may not be there, a job of an equivalent nature must be offered.

Types of work

It is an implicit and undiscussed assumption (by men) that any woman who works outside the home will continue to keep house as well. Hence housework must always be considered when examining work in pregnancy. All women work in the

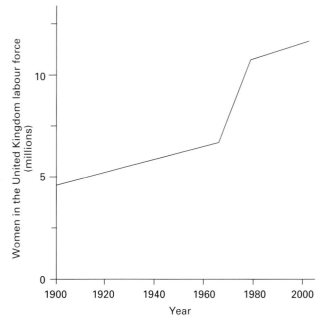

Figure 6.1 Numbers of women in the labour force in the UK

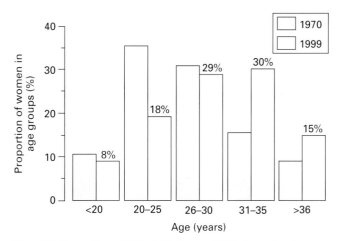

Figure 6.2 Proportions of births in England and Wales by maternal age in 1970 and 1999

Box 6.1   Current maternity benefits (April 2001)

Statutory maternity pay (from employer)
- Non-contributory
- Taxable
- Overlapping
- Paid for 18 weeks—90% of wage for first 6 weeks, £62.20 a week thereafter

Maternity allowance (from DSS)
- Contributory
- Taxable
- Paid for 18 weeks at £62.20 per week

Sure/Start Maternity grant (from DSS)
- £300

Maternity leave
- 18 weeks (see text)

house, where there is washing, cooking, cleaning, and the loads imposed by other children, a husband, and maybe parents. When a woman works at home she has no rest or meal breaks; if she works outside the home as well, housework is often done in the evenings and at weekends.

About 45% of jobs done by women are part time so, although the activity may be great, the number of hours spent away from the home are fewer.

Specific hazards at work

Outside the home three million women work in offices, two million in hotels and shops, and one million in the health service or education; another four million work in a wide range of jobs, though few women in this country do the very heavy jobs that are done by women in the United States and the former Soviet Union, for example. Indeed, in this country under the Mines Act 1889 women are not allowed to work down mines.

Most women are aware of specific hazards in their workplace. These are most important in very early pregnancy, when teratogenic influences may occur at a specific time in embryogenesis. The same stimulus acting later in pregnancy can affect growth, causing intrauterine growth restriction.

Chemical hazards

Over 30 000 individual chemicals are used in industry, with a further 3000 compounds being added each year. It is impossible to test all of them on pregnant animals, and much of the evidence about safety depends on retrospective reports of damage to humans. The number of chemicals that are proved to be teratogenic are few.

If a woman is worried about chemicals in her workplace and consults her family doctor, the doctor would do well to discuss the problem with a health and safety officer or trade union official at the woman's work. If there is no help there, the best reference source is the local or central office of the Health and Safety Executive. Any woman who thinks that she is working with a toxic hazard should discuss this well before pregnancy for it is often too late to start making enquiries in early pregnancy. There are special codes of practice for certain toxic chemicals which safeguard pregnant women and their unborn children. The employer should offer alternative work with no loss of pay or benefits. Toxic chemicals can still enter the mother's body after childbirth and be excreted in milk, so a lactating mother also should take precautions against such chemicals.

Many chemicals have been blamed at some time for affecting an early embryo. This makes big news but when, a few years later, the reports are refuted, it is not newsworthy and often not reported in newspapers.

Box 6.2 Chemical hazards in pregnancy
- Metals—for example, lead, mercury, copper
- Gases—for example, carbon monoxide
- Passive smoking
- Insecticides
- Herbicides
- Solvents—for example, carbon tetrachloride
- Drugs during their manufacture
- Disinfecting agents—for example, ethylene oxide

Physical hazards

At specific times in embryogenesis physical hazards can cause abnormalities. X rays are a risk in early pregnancy, particularly if a series of films of abdominal structures are exposed during

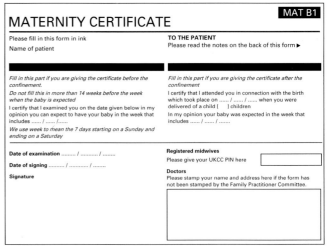

Figure 6.3 Maternity certificate

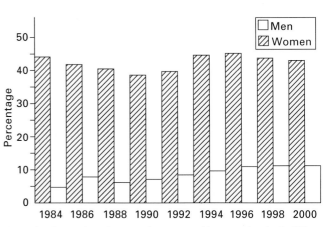

Figure 6.4 Proportion of men and women working part time in the UK

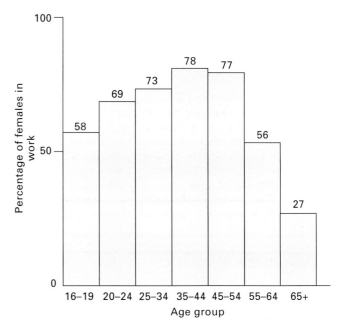

Figure 6.5 Female economic workforce by age

early pregnancy, e.g. for intravenous urography or barium studies of the intestine. It is wise always to ask about the last menstrual period, contraceptive practices, and the possibility of pregnancy specifically before any *x* ray in women of childbearing age. The 10-day rule (whereby no woman is exposed to *x* rays within 10 days of the next menstrual period) has now lapsed in most hospitals but inquiry should be made.

The risks of *x* rays to the female staff in a well managed therapeutic radiation department are probably low, but some women work with radioisotopes in laboratories. The Health and Safety Executive has laid down standards that women should follow. Less well regulated are the *x* ray machines used for security checks in many large firms. There is probably little risk to a visitor passing once through the system, but the people who work the equipment might be exposed to repeated radiation, which should be checked.

Ultrasound is used widely in industry and at the dosage used is probably safe. Certainly, diagnostic ultrasound used in medicine has low energy and is pulsatile; the risk of cell damage or vacuolation that occurs with high energy ultrasound does not exist with this common use. There is no epidemiological evidence of medical ultrasound associated abnormalities: some 60 million women have been exposed to ultrasound in early pregnancy, yet no pattern of problems has yet been shown. Nearly all pregnant women in the UK have one or two ultrasound scans but 46% report having more than two during the pregnancy.

Another physical hazard which caused a scare was the use of visual display units (VDUs) in personal computers (PCs). There are millions of PCs in the homes and offices of the UK. Some 20 years ago small groups of women working with VDUs were reported to have a high rate of pregnancy wastage. These were small clusters, and the measured outcomes were often a mixture of miscarriage, congenital abnormality, and stillbirth. More recent studies show no increased risk due to the use of such units and a wide ranging review concluded, "At present it seems reasonable to conclude that pregnancy will not be harmed by using the VDU. Statements on the contrary are not soundly based."[1]

Biological hazards

Nurses, female doctors, and others who handle body fluids, as well as women who work in microbiological laboratories may be handling toxic materials, but usage is usually well regulated for all workers in or out of pregnancy. Rules must be followed.

Animal workers may be at increased risk, and there have been reports of miscarriage after handling ewes at lambing because of the passage of ovine chlamydia, and toxoplasmosis infection may be more prevalent among those who handle domestic pets in their jobs. The position with bovine spongiform encephalopathy (BSE) for pregnant workers is unclear for too few cases have been documented. There is probably no extra risk over background for the pregnant.

Probably the most commonly transmitted infection which may affect the fetus is German measles. Epidemics occur among young children, and so teachers who are constantly in contact with them are at risk. All young women entering teaching should have their serum rubella antibody titre checked; if they are found to be seronegative they should be offered vaccination.

Non-specific hazards

As well as specified toxins, various physiological changes of pregnancy in the mother might affect the embryo deleteriously. During strenuous exercise the blood supply to the non-skeletal parts of the body are reduced, including the kidneys, intestines,

Box 6.3   Physical hazards in pregnancy
- Ionising radiation—for example, *x* rays
- Noise
- Vibration
- Heat
- Humidity
- Repetitive muscular work—for example, at visual display units
- Lifting heavy loads
- Uninterrupted standing

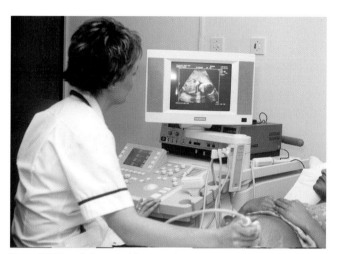

Figure 6.6 Use of ultrasound for screening

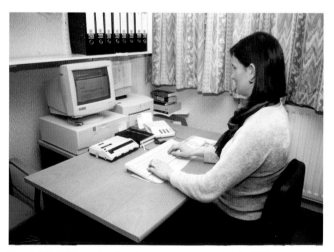

Figure 6.7 Millions of personal computers are used in the UK

Normal pregnant women in jobs with no toxic risk need not be deterred from working for as long as they wish into pregnancy.

Box 6.4   Biological hazards in pregnancy
- Contact in crowded places—for example, in travelling to work
- Contact with higher risk group—for example, schoolchildren
- Food preparation
- Waterborne infections
- New arrivals from abroad

and uterus; the blood supply to the leg muscles can be increased 20-fold and that to the uterus halved. Hence in hard physical work, as occurs in agriculture, there may be some diminution of uterine blood flow, but this is unlikely with ordinary work. Similarly, stress can reduce blood flow to the uterus if the degree of agitation is high enough; if a woman is working inside her own limits there probably will be no problem.

Environmental factors at work that induce boredom and fatigue were found to have effects on pregnant women in a French study.[2] Women in industrial and agricultural jobs were compared with those working in offices. Multivariant analyses of the repetitive nature of the work, the physical effort required, the boredom of the work, standing, and the effect of background noise showed an increased proportion of preterm deliveries when these factors were high, and this might be important in women who have previously had preterm labours.

Recent British and U.S. studies found no effect of work on birth weight.[3] Infants born to women in full-time employment had no significant differences from those born to women who were not in paid work. Data on hours of work, energy expenditure, and posture were collected at 17, 28, and 36 weeks, and these too had no discernible association with birth weight.

It is probable that a higher proportion of those who work are well women and those with chronic ill health do not work. (Further, those of better educational attainments report more out of home work than those with less.) Nevertheless, once the sociobiological variables are removed, work in pregnancy is still associated with a better outcome.

Travel to work

If a woman has paid work outside the home, she has to get there. If travelling entails a short walk in the morning and evening it can be enjoyable, but most women live in large towns with an unpleasant 30–90 minutes of travel at the beginning and end of the day. There is noise, heat, fatigue, and, in some cases, other people's tobacco smoke. Travel is stressful in crowded, unpleasant conditions. Studies in Spain showed that the likelihood of preterm labour increases with the duration of stressful public travel the woman has to suffer.[4] It may be wise for a woman contemplating pregnancy to arrange to work flexible hours if her work is in a big city. The employer could then perhaps allow her to arrive a little before or after the rush hour, with time being made up in other ways.

Conclusion

More women work during pregnancy and want to continue for longer. Pregnancy is a normal event and, generally speaking, most jobs cause no increased hazard to the mother or baby. A woman should, however, be warned that if any complications arise she must be able to leave work easily. If there is flexibility and the job is not one entailing a high risk from toxic agents most women can continue working for as long as they wish in pregnancy.

When the effects of work on maternal and fetal outcomes are assessed, after adjusting for environmental and background social factors, work seems to have very little detrimental or beneficial influence.

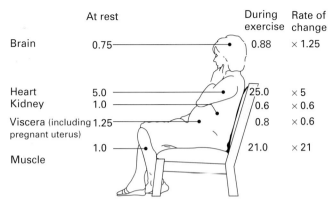

Figure 6.8 Changes in blood flow (l/min) in pregnancy, at rest and during exercise

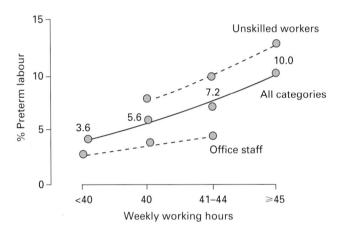

Figure 6.9 Weekly working hours and rate of preterm labour

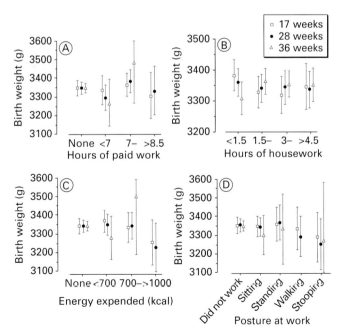

Figure 6.10 Birth weight and work. An antenatal population was sampled at 17, 28, and 36 weeks of gestation[3]

References

1 Blackwell R, Chang A. Video display terminals and pregnancy. *Br J Obstet Gynaec* 1988;**95**:446–53.
2 Mamelle N, Laumon B. Occupational fatigue and preterm birth. In: Chamberlain G, ed. *Pregnant women at work*. London: Royal Society of Medicine, 1984;105–16.
3 Rabkin CS, Anderson HR, Bland JM, Brooke OG, Peacock JL, Chamberlain G. Maternal activity and birthweight. *Am J Epidemiol* 1990;**131**:522–31.
4 Rodrigues-Escudero R, Belanstegreguria A, Gutierrez-Martinez S. Perinatal complications of work and pregnancy. *An Esp Pediatr* 1980;**13**:465–76.

Recommended reading

● Chamberlain G. Work in pregnancy. *Am J Indust Med* 1993;**23**:559–75.
● Henriksen T, Savitz D, Hedegaard M, Secher N. Employment during pregnancy in relation to risk factors and pregnancy outcome. *Br J Obstet Gynaec* 1994;**101**:858–65.
● Maternity Alliance. Factsheets on allowances and benefits in pregnancy. London: Maternity Alliance, 2001.

The form MATB1 has Crown copyright and is reproduced by permission of the Controller of Her Majesty's Stationery Office. The figure showing weekly working hours is reproduced with permission from Office for National Statistics. *Labour force survey* 1984–2000. London: ONS, 2001.

7 Vaginal bleeding in early pregnancy

Bleeding drives patients to their general practitioner swiftly. Vaginal bleeding early in pregnancy makes the woman think that she may be miscarrying, so this brings her even more promptly; the practitioner thence has the opportunity to diagnose the cause and start management.

Bleeding has four known causes in early pregnancy (Box 7.1). In addition, bleeding may occur for no apparent reason in a large number of cases. In early pregnancy such cases are commonly categorised as threatened miscarriage, but this is fudging the issue for in many cases the conceptus and its future placental system are not involved; doctors should be honest and say that they do not know the cause rather than mislabel it.

Miscarriage and abortion

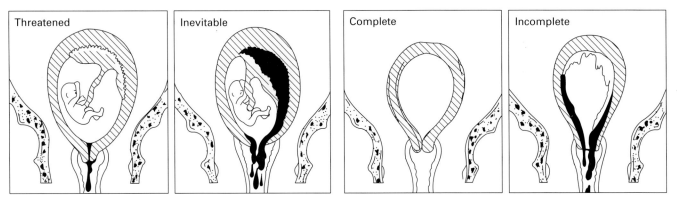

Figure 7.1 In a *threatened* miscarriage the cervix is still closed and there is not much bleeding. In an *inevitable* miscarriage the cervix has started to open and the membranes often have ruptured. There is usually more bleeding. A *complete* miscarriage means that the uterus is empty of clot and decidua. In an *incomplete* miscarriage the embryo has been passed vaginally but some part of the membrane or decidua is retained. There may also be clots

The terms miscarriage and abortion have been used synonymously but miscarriage is the word which should be associated with the spontaneous event.

- *Threatened miscarriage.* Women bleed a little from the vagina during a threatened miscarriage but there is not much abdominal pain. The uterus is enlarged and the cervix closed. Pregnancy may continue.
- *Inevitable miscarriage.* Miscarriage is inevitable if the cervical os is open. Blood loss can be great and lower abdominal cramping pains accompany the uterine contractions. Some products of conception and clots may be passed but often decidua is retained and then the miscarriage is called incomplete.
- *Complete miscarriage.* The cervical os is open and the uterus completely expels its contents. Such miscarriages are more likely after 14 weeks of pregnancy than earlier, when they are often incomplete.
- *Septic miscarriage.* This follows the ascent of organisms from the vagina into the uterus, often after an incomplete miscarriage or an induced abortion under non-sterile conditions. As well as heavy bleeding and pain, the woman commonly has a fever and may develop signs of endotoxic shock. The commonest organisms are *Escherichia coli* and *Streptococcus faecalis*.
- *Silent miscarriage.* The embryo dies and is eventually absorbed but the uterus does not expel the decidua and sac of membranes. The woman sometimes feels a dull weight in

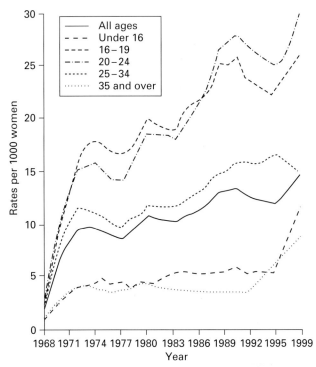

Figure 7.2 Terminations of pregnancy by age group in England and Wales, 1968–99. Many operations are performed outside the NHS, some being done through charity clinics

the pelvis, the symptoms of pregnancy regress and the uterus stops enlarging. Old blood is passed as a brown, watery discharge. This condition is diagnosed more frequently now that ultrasonography is used in very early pregnancy.

● *Recurrent miscarriage* is diagnosed when a woman has three or more consecutive spontaneous miscarriages. Such women deserve gynaecological and immunological investigation; many gynaecologists start investigations after two consecutive miscarriages in women over 35. A specific cause for the recurrence can be found in up to 40% of cases.

● *Therapeutic abortion*. This is now common in Britain, with over 180 000 women in England and Wales having such abortions each year. Usually the general practitioner knows but occasionally the woman has bypassed him, presenting only after the event with vaginal bleeding, an open cervix, and some abdominal pain. This means that decidua or blood clot is left in the uterus and needs the same attention as does an incomplete miscarriage.

Causes of miscarriage

Embryonic abnormalities
Chromosomal abnormalities are common, arising from a change in the nucleus of either gamete or a spontaneous mutation inside the fertilised oocyte. At the time of fertilisation splitting and rejoining of genetic material may be imperfect. Such changes are not usually recurrent, and parents should be told this.

Immunological rejection
The fetus is genetically foreign to the mother and yet most fetuses are not rejected. In many cases blocking antibodies that inhibit the cell-mediated rejection of the embryo are stimulated by antigens from the trophoblast. Antiphospholipid antibodies have been linked with recurrent early pregnancy loss as well as later placental bed insufficiency. This may act through placental thrombosis or decidual vasculopathy. Treatment with aspirin, heparin or a combination offers hope of a successful pregnancy.

Uterine abnormalities
The uterus is formed during embryonic development from two tubes fusing together to make a common cavity. Occasionally various degrees of non-absorption in the midline septum occur, leaving either two cavities or a cavity partly divided by a septum down the middle. The blood supply to this median structure is usually poor and implantation of an embryo here may be followed by miscarriage.

Cervical incompetence
The cervix may have some weakness which could be associated with a spontaneous miscarriage in the mid-trimester (13–27 weeks). This can be either congenital or acquired after overstretching at a previous dilatation and curettage or birth. The unsupported membranes bulge into the cervical canal through the internal os and rupture early, which causes the abortive process. The incompetence may be diagnosed before pregnancy by a hysterogram (a radiological examination of the uterine cavity) or in pregnancy by ultrasonography. Cervical cerclage is usually performed in pregnancy following a history of mid-trimester miscarriage, particularly if the membranes ruptured before any uterine contractions occurred (see Chapter 12).

Maternal disease
This is unlikely to be a major cause of miscarriage in the UK, but hypertension and renal disease are still associated with

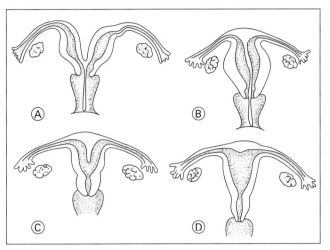

Figure 7.3 Congenital abnormalities of the uterus caused by non-absorption of the septum during fusion of the Müllerian ducts. (A) Complete double uterus, double cervix, and vaginal septum. (B) Double uterine cavity within a single body; the cervix and the vagina have a septum. (C) A subseptate uterus in which the septum does not reach down to the cervix. (D) Arcuate uterus with a dimple on top of the single uterus with a single cervix

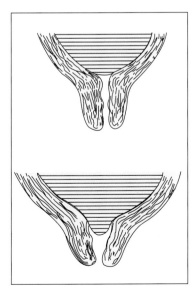

Figure 7.4 Above: normal cervix with maternal os closed protecting amniotic sac. Below: incompetent internal cervical os with membranes bulging

higher rates of miscarriage in later pregnancy. Maternal infections can affect the fetus, particularly rubella, toxoplasmosis, cytomegalic inclusion disease, and listeriosis. Severe maternal malnutrition is most unusual in this country, though it can still occur in developing countries. Deficiency of individual vitamins (such as vitamin E) is extraordinarily rare in the mixed diet of this country, and there is no evidence of it being a substantial cause of miscarriage in women. Shortage of folic acid is associated with fetuses with major central nervous system abnormalities, some of which may miscarry.

Endocrine imbalance

Diabetes and thyroid hyperfunction are associated with increased risks of spontaneous miscarriage. If diagnosed, both are now usually well controlled and the risk is reduced. Abnormalities in the ratio of luteinising hormone to follicle-stimulating hormone in a particular cycle may lead to miscarriage. An insufficiency of progesterone from the corpus luteum used to be regarded as a cause of miscarriage. This is hard to prove, and most randomised trials using progestogens in early pregnancy have failed to show an improvement. Some consider that hCG injections may help. If, however, the woman has faith in this treatment and had a previous successful pregnancy taking it, the practitioner would do well to treat the psyche as well as the soma and prescribe a progestogen or hCG.

Criminal abortion

This is now much less common in Britain but still occurs in other countries and in populations derived from those countries. Although infection has been introduced, only rarely do criminal abortionists leave signs that can be spotted in the genital tract and so the woman is often treated for an incomplete or septic miscarriage. With the reduction in illegal abortion, maternal mortality from this cause has disappeared in the UK.

Presentation

A woman who is miscarrying usually presents with vaginal bleeding and may have some low abdominal pain. The bleeding is slight in a threatened miscarriage, greater amounts being present with an inevitable miscarriage. Pain with uterine contractions may be compared with dysmenorrhoea. The degree of shock usually relates to the amount of blood loss from the body and the degree of cervical dilatation.

The differential diagnosis includes ectopic pregnancy and salpingitis.

Management

Threatened miscarriage

A woman with a threatened miscarriage is best removed from an active environment. If the practitioner tells her to go to bed to rest for 48 hours she may feel happier but there is no real evidence that bedrest makes any difference to the incidence of miscarriage. Some 5% of women who deliver safely report vaginal bleeding in the same pregnancy; the effectiveness of specific treatments is difficult to assess. The avoidance of sexual intercourse is probably sensible as it might act as a local stimulus.

Inevitable miscarriage

If events progress to an inevitable miscarriage the woman often needs to be assessed in hospital;[1] an ecbolic agent might be

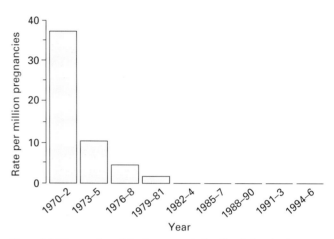

Figure 7.5 The number of deaths reported after illegal abortion is reducing rapidly in England and Wales, with none reported for the 14 years 1982–96. Death used to be mostly from sepsis or renal or hepatic failure

Box 7.3	Treatment of miscarriage
Threatened	Bedrest
	Avoid intercourse
	Reassure with ultrasound
Inevitable	Hospitalisation
	If heavy bleeding, use ecbolic
	Evacuate uterus

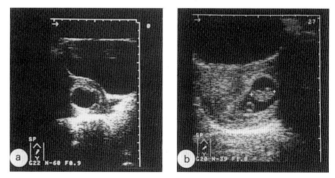

Figure 7.6 (A) Ultrasound scan of an empty sac in the uterus at seven weeks gestation. This woman had a silent miscarriage, the embryo having been resorbed. (B) Ultrasound scan of a continuing pregnancy at just over seven weeks; fetal tissue is easily seen between the crosses

given if the bleeding is excessive and a paramedic may be needed to cover transfer. Ultrasound is useful in determining if the miscarriage is complete. Retained products can be removed surgically under a general anaesthetic or medically using vaginal prostaglandins.

Complete miscarriage

This is more common than was once thought; practitioners may see the sac containing the embryo and feel that this is complete. They would do well to remember, however, that a large amount of decidua can be left behind and an evacuation may prevent the woman having a haemorrhage or infection a week or so later. Ultrasound in an early pregnancy unit can help to make the diagnosis.

Silent miscarriage

This is sometimes diagnosed from the woman's symptoms of a brown discharge and a heavy, dull feeling in the pelvis; the finding of no embryonic tissue inside the gestation sac on ultrasonography confirms the diagnosis. It can also appear as a complete surprise at a routine ultrasound. Management options include a conservative line with a repeat ultrasound, surgical evacuation or medical management with prostaglandins.

Septic abortion

This may require the full management of severe sepsis. Endocervical swabs should be sent to the laboratory and treatment with a broad spectrum antibiotic started immediately. Central venous pressure measurement and intravenous rehydration will be required; the urinary output should be watched carefully. Evidence of disseminated intravascular coagulopathy should be sought and the uterus evacuated once a reasonable tissue concentration of antibiotics has been achieved. Watch for renal failure.

Recurrent miscarriage

The management of recurrent abortion is outside the scope of this series but some aetiological features are given in Box 7.1. It requires sympathetic handling by both general practitioners and specialists.

Ectopic pregnancy

An ectopic pregnancy is one that implants and develops outside the uterine cavity. The sites are shown in the figure, but most (96%) are in the fallopian tube.

Causes

Anything that slows the passage of the fertilised oocyte down the fallopian tube can cause a tubal ectopic pregnancy. Previous tubal infection, an intrauterine device in place, and late fertilisation are quoted causes, but in most ectopic pregnancies no cause is found.

Presentation

A tubal ectopic pregnancy may either rupture through the wall (more common with isthmial and cornual implantations) or leak a little blood from the lateral end of the fallopian tube (with ampullary or fimbrial implantations). Vaginal bleeding can occur.

With rupture there is a brisk peritoneal reaction and the woman may fall to the ground as though kicked in the stomach.

Box 7.4   Treatment of severe septic abortion

- **Hypovolaemia**
  - Monitor—Blood pressure
    - Central venous pressure
    - Cardiac output
    - Renal output
  - Treatment—Intravenous rehydration and maintenance
- **Infection**
  - Identify organisms
  - Treatment—Systemic
    - Antibodies
    - —Local
      - Evacuate uterus (dilatation and curettage)
      - Remove uterus (hysterectomy)
- **Coagulation abnormalities**
- **Renal shutdown**
  - Monitor oliguria
  - Monitor electrolytes
  - Plan early dialysis
  - Watch for renal failure
- **Respiratory system**
  - Monitor—Blood gases
  - Treatment—Oxygen
    - Ventilate
- **Anaemia and white cell deficiencies**

Table 7.1 Current aetiological causes of recurrent miscarriage

Cause	Major manifestations
Anatomical	Uterine cavity anomalies, cervical incompetence
Infective	Bacterial vaginitis
Genetic	Incorrect implanting of genome
Endocrine	Defective corpus luteum, luteal phase deficiency
Autoimmune	Systemic lupus erythematosus, antiphospholipid syndrome
No obvious cause is found by current tests in 30% of all cases	

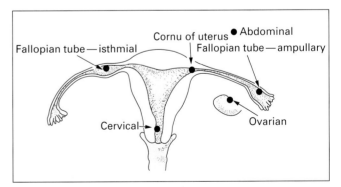

Figure 7.7 Possible sites for ectopic pregnancy

She quickly becomes very shocked because of the large volume of blood released into the peritoneal cavity and the stimulation of the peritoneum. The abdomen is tender with guarding and rebound tenderness, and vaginal examination causes intense pain on touching the cervix.

A more gradual leak from the tubal end causes irritation of the pouch of Douglas. The woman goes to her doctor complaining of vague, low abdominal pain, sometimes with vaginal bleeding occurring after the pain. The abdomen may be uncomfortable in the suprapubic area, and a very gentle vaginal assessment may show a tenderness in the pouch of Douglas or in the adnexa on one side.

The differential diagnosis includes an abortion or any other cause for a sudden release of blood into the peritoneal cavity, such as a bleeding vessel over an ovarian cyst. Inflammatory conditions such as appendicitis may mimic a leaking ectopic pregnancy. Ectopic pregnancy should always be considered in any cases of lower abdominal pain because an unruptured ectopic pregnancy, leaking a little blood over the course of some days, is hard to diagnose. A negative routine pregnancy test is not exclusive; it is usually positive.

Management

The management of a woman with a ruptured ectopic pregnancy is straightforward. She should go to hospital immediately, if necessary accompanied by her general practitioner. Intravenous support may be required in the home, and in severe cases a flying squad (if available) may be required. Once in the hospital, surgery should be immediate. Most tubal ectopic pregnancies need a laparoscopy to confirm the diagnosis and maybe provide access for treatment. Those in severe shock due to a ruptured ectopic will also need a laparotomy and surgical removal. Unruptured ectopics can be managed laparoscopically by opening the tube and aspirating the gestational material. If some part of the tube can be left behind it is psychologically helpful to the woman. There is a small risk of a second ectopic pregnancy developing in the remaining tube but there is also the possibility of reparative surgery later. This is particularly important when a woman has had a previous ectopic pregnancy and one fallopian tube has already been removed.

A leaking tubal pregnancy is harder to diagnose, such cases being usually referred to outpatient departments in a more leisurely fashion. If the diagnosis is suspected, laparoscopy is the best test; ultrasonography is not exclusive, although fluid in the pouch of Douglas with no intrauterine pregnancy in a woman with 6–8 weeks' amenorrhoea and a raised hCG level is highly suggestive.[2] At laparoscopy the swollen area of the tube can usually be seen and little blood may come from the lateral end. Under ultrasound guidance, injections of fetotoxic agents such as methotrexate or potassium chloride are given. Alternatively, some, having made a firm diagnosis of ectopic pregnancy by a raised hCG, an empty uterus, and ultrasound evidence of fluid in the pouch of Douglas, will treat the woman conservatively if the ectopic is unruptured. Systemic methotrexate given as a single dose works in 90%. If hCG levels persist, a second dose a few days later usually suffices. The results of such minimally invasive management are as good as those of more conservative surgery, with the time spent in hospital and the emotional effects on the woman's life being much reduced.

> **Any woman treated for an ectopic pregnancy should be warned of the increased chances of a recurrence. The increased risk is said to be seven times above background.**

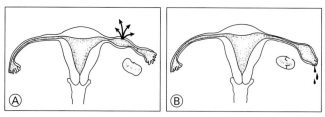

Figure 7.8 The most common ectopic pregnancies are in the fallopian tube. (A) Those at the medial end rupture. (B) Those at the lateral end leak more gradually

Table 7.2 Symptoms and signs of ectopic pregnancy

	Unruptured	Ruptured
Symptoms	Gradual onset	Sudden onset
	Dull ache over days	Severe pain over minutes
Signs	No shock	Commonly shocked
	Vague suprapubic tenderness	Rigid abdomen with rebound tenderness
	No great cervical tenderness	Extreme tenderness on cervical movement
	Vague mass often felt	Too tender to palpate

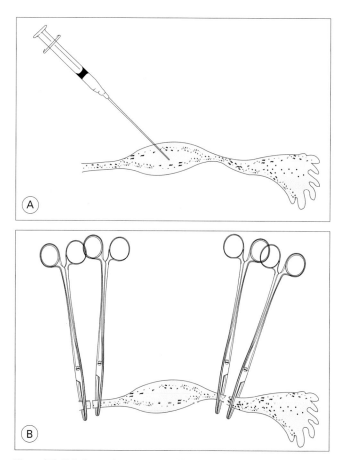

Figure 7.9 Tubal ectopic pregnancy. (A) Laparoscopic injection of methotrexate, a fetocidal substance. (B) Clamping and cutting out of the affected part of the tube at open surgery

Gestational trophoblastic disease

Causes

Chromosomal changes in the fertilised oocyte lead to degeneration of the stem blood vessels in the villi in very early pregnancy, so producing a vast overgrowth of swollen villae (vesicles) inside the uterus. This is a hydatidiform mole, and commonly no embryo is found. It is usually benign but in less than 10% of cases it develops into an invasive mole or even a gestational choriocarcinoma.

Although rare in the UK (0·6 per 1000 pregnancies), hydatidiform moles and their malignant sequelae seem to be reported more commonly in other parts of the world such as in the Pacific region (2·0 per 1000 pregnancies).

Presentation

A woman with a mole will bleed, sometimes heavily, after 6–8 weeks of gestation. She is often unwell with signs of anaemia and excessive vomiting. Proteinuric hypertension can occur as early as eight weeks. After 12 weeks of gestation the uterus often feels much bigger than expected for dates but no fetal parts can be felt or fetal heart heard. Occasionally the woman may pass vesicles through the vagina; this is diagnostic but rarely occurs.

Moles are diagnosed from this clinical presentation backed up by either an excessively high estimation of human chorionic gonadotrophin in the urine or by ultrasonography, when a characteristic picture is seen.

The differential diagnosis must include twins with a threatened miscarriage, but ultrasonography, which should be readily available to most general practitioners, gives the answer immediately.

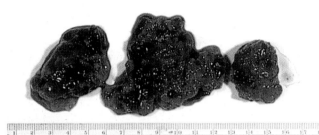

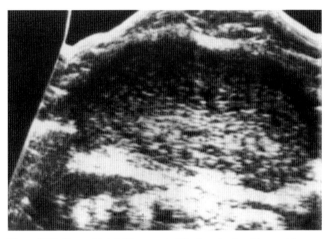

Figure 7.10 Above: Hydatidiform mole. The bunch of vesicles rapidly expands the uterine cavity. Below: A hydatidiform mole may be diagnosed readily on ultrasonography, the sound waves being reflected off the vesicles to give a picture of soap bubble foam. With early ultrasound equipment, however, hydatidiform moles looked like a snowstorm and so this term came into use. Do not expect snow if you use a B scan machine, the now commonly used apparatus

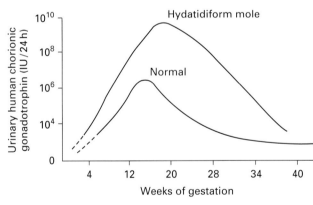

Figure 7.11 Human chorionic gonadotrophin values are much higher in women with a hydatidiform mole than in women with a normal pregnancy (note the log scale on the y-axis)

Management

Once diagnosed a mole should be evacuated quickly. The woman should be admitted to hospital and a suction curettage performed under anaesthesia with the protection of an oxytocin drip. All tissue is sent to the laboratory for examination of its neoplastic potential.

After an evacuation all women should be registered for follow up at one of the supraregional trophoblast disease centres, where human chorionic gonadotrophin concentrations in urine or blood can be measured. If these are high at six weeks chemotherapy is recommended to prevent subsequent malignancy.

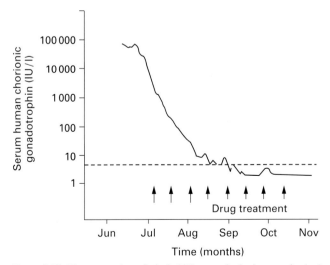

Figure 7.12 After evacuation of a hydatidiform mole the human chorionic gonadotrophin concentration remains high. Methotrexate and folinic acid were given on nine occasions, the treatment being associated with a reduction in hormone concentration

Other causes of vaginal bleeding

Bleeding may come from local problems in the vagina or cervix.

- Cervical ectropion is common in pregnancy; bleeding is not profuse.
- Vaginal or cervical infections can cause mild bleeding.
- Adenomas and polyps of the cervix become more pronounced during pregnancy. They may bleed on stimulation.
- Carcinoma of the cervix is rare but important in women of childbearing age. It may cause bleeding on stimulation and examination with a speculum reveals the cause. If there is any doubt a biopsy must be performed under anaesthesia even when a woman is pregnant.
- A general maternal disease such as blood dysplasia, von Willebrand's disease, or leukaemia may cause symptoms in rare cases.

Lesions of the cervix or vagina may cause bleeding in early pregnancy.

References

1 Westergaard J, Teisner B, Sinosich M *et al.* Ultrasound and biochemical tests in the prediction of early pregnancy failure. *Br J Obstet Gynaec* 1985;**92**:77–83.
2 Cacciatore B, Stenman U, Yostalo P. Diagnosis of ectopic pregnancy. *Br J Obstet Gynaec* 1990;**97**:904–8.

Recommended reading

- Aukum W. Diagnosing suspected ectopic pregnancy. *Br Med J* 2000;**321**:1235–60.
- Hejenius P. Interventions for tubal ectopic pregnancy. Cochrane Database of Systematic Reviews. Oxford: Update Software, 2000.
- Kulteh W. Recurrent pregnancy loss—an update. *Curr Opin Obstet Gynaec* 1999;**11**:904–8.
- Rai R, Regan L. Obstetric complications of antiphospholipid antibodies syndrome. *Curr Opin Obstet Gynaec* 1997;**9**:387–390.
- RCOG. *Management of gestational trophoblast disease.* Guidelines no. 18. London: RCOG, 1999.

8 Antenatal medical and surgical problems

Pregnant women are usually young and fit. They rarely have chronic medical conditions but when they do, those in charge of antenatal care need to consider how the disease might affect pregnancy and how pregnancy might affect the disease.

Heart disease

Most heart disease in women of childbearing age is rheumatic in origin despite the recent great reduction in the prevalence of rheumatic fever. Better living conditions in the UK and the more prompt treatment of streptococcal sore throats with antibiotics in childhood have reduced rheumatic damage to the heart valves and myocardium. An increasing proportion of pregnant women have congenital heart lesions that have been treated previously.

Pregnancy puts an increased load on the cardiovascular system. More blood has to be circulated so that cardiac output increases by up to 40% by mid-pregnancy, staying steady until labour, when it increases further. This increased cardiac work cannot be done as effectively by a damaged heart; if the heart is compromised a woman would be wise to avoid other increased loads that might precipitate cardiac failure. The most frequently encountered are:

- Household work
- Paid work outside the home
- Care of other family members
- Pre-eclampsia
- Anaemia
- Recrudescence of rheumatic fever
- Respiratory infection
- Urinary infection
- Bacterial endocarditis

Care should be taken just after delivery: with the uterine retraction up to a litre of blood can be swiftly shunted from the uterine veins into the general venous system.

Rheumatic heart disease
The commonest single cardiac lesion found in women of this age group is rheumatic mitral stenosis, sometimes accompanied by the after effects of rheumatic myocarditis. The commonest complication of overload is pulmonary oedema in late pregnancy or immediately after delivery. Right-sided cardiac failure may occur but is less common.

Cardiomyopathy of pregnancy occurs mostly post partum but occasionally in late pregnancy. There is no obvious predisposing cause; the heart is greatly distorted, leading to right-sided cardiac failure.

Congenital lesions
The most serious of the congenital lesions in pregnancy are those accompanied by shunts.

- Women with Eisenmenger's syndrome do particularly badly in pregnancy, especially those with severe pulmonary hypertension, which leads to a right to left shunt.
- Tetralogy of Fallot has a lower risk of cardiac failure because there is less resistance at the pulmonary valve regulating right ventricular outflow.
- Artificial heart valves are now present in an increasing number of women who become pregnant. Commonly they are man-made replacements of the mitral or aortic valve; affected women continue anticoagulant treatment with warfarin despite the theoretical risk of teratogenesis in early

Box 8.1   Problem diseases in pregnancy
- Heart disease
- Diabetes
- Thyroid disease
- Epilepsy
- Jaundice
- Anaemia
- Haemoglobinopathies
- Urinary tract infection
- HIV infection
- Psychiatric changes and diseases

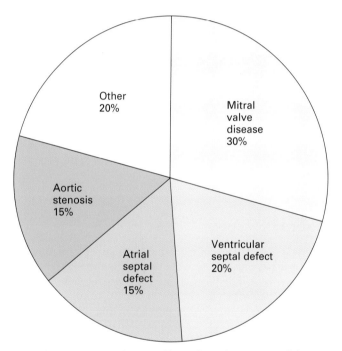

Figure 8.1 Main structural causes of heart disease in pregnancy. Other causes of heart disease include thyrotoxicosis and coronary artery disease

Table 8.1   Modified New York Heart Association's classification of exercise tolerance

	Symptoms of cardiac insufficiency	Limitation of activities
I	None	None
II	Only after exercise	With moderate exercise
III	After any activity	With ordinary activities
IV	At rest	Unable to perform any physical activities

pregnancy and fetal bleeding later. It is still widely used and may be replaced two or three weeks before the expected date of delivery by heparin.

Management

Most women with heart disease who are of childbearing age are known to their family practitioner. He or she should ensure that they go for antenatal care at a centre where a cardiologist works alongside an obstetrician, ideally at a combined cardiac antenatal clinic if there are enough cases.

Early assessment should be made of the severity of the disease, paying attention to the features that may worsen the prognosis: the woman's age, the severity of the lesion, the type of lesion, and the degree of decompensation (exercise tolerance). Rest should be encouraged during pregnancy and extra physical loads avoided. Labour should be booked at a consultant unit with an interested cardiologist involved. The ward may need the extra drugs and equipment to be available if a woman with a heart condition is admitted. Delivery should be planned at a unit with ready access to a cardiac centre and availability of cardiologists and cardiac anaesthetists.

Care should be taken to avoid the development of acute bacterial endocarditis by ensuring that the woman is given antibiotics when she has any infection or is at potential risk of developing an infection—for example, at a tooth extraction or labour. This precaution is more important for congenital lesions of the heart than for rheumatic lesions.

The prognosis for a woman with heart disease in pregnancy is now greatly improved. It used inevitably to be associated with deterioration of the heart condition, but now, with proper care, this is not so.

Diabetes

Diabetes is a metabolic disease found in about 1% of women of childbearing age. In addition, another 1–2% of women will develop gestational diabetes during the course of their pregnancy; the incidence is higher in older than younger women. Glycosuria (checked by dipstick testing) is even more common than this, occurring at some time in pregnancy in up to 15% of women and is no longer a screening test for diabetes in pregnancy. Instead finger-prick or venous blood samples should be checked for blood sugar levels.

Established insulin dependent diabetes

Four fifths of women with diabetes are known to the practitioner before they become pregnant. All diabetic women of reproductive age should be using effective contraception and be encouraged to attend a prepregnancy clinic so that pregnancy is planned. Good control of diabetes before and in early pregnancy reduces the incidence of congenital anomalies and miscarriage.

Antenatal care is best performed by an obstetrician and a diabetic physician at a combined diabetic antenatal clinic. The general practitioner must be kept well informed of changes in management of the diabetes during pregnancy, because between antenatal clinic visits the woman may depend on her family practitioner for continuity of care. Detailed ultrasonography to exclude congenital abnormalities and to monitor growth is vital.

Pregnancy makes the control of diabetes more difficult; close monitoring is the key to a successful outcome. Women are encouraged to eat enough carbohydrate to satisfy them without

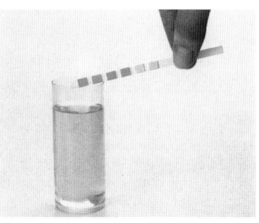

Box 8.2   Drugs which may be needed when a woman with severe heart disease is admitted in pregnancy or labour
- Oxygen
- Digoxin
- Frusemide
- Aminophylline

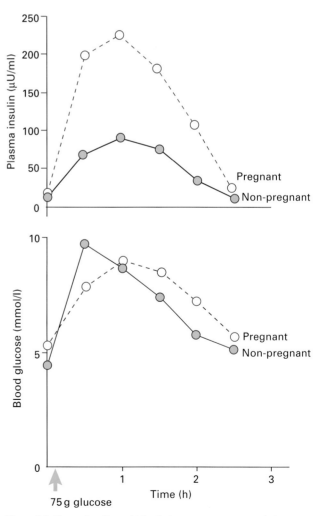

Figure 8.2 Dipstick testing of urine

Figure 8.3 Plasma insulin and blood glucose response to oral glucose (75 g) in pregnant and non-pregnant women

restriction and should take regular snacks between meals. Most women who have attended a prepregnancy clinic will have already been converted to a basal bolus insulin regime. This consists of three short-acting doses during the day and one long-acting insulin dose at night. This regime enables good glucose control to be achieved and is started in early pregnancy, if not before.

Glucose concentrations in blood are measured by the woman as frequently as four times a day with her own glucose meter at home. Virtually all diabetic women require an increase in their insulin dosage during pregnancy. Frequent clinic visits are necessary to facilitate this and the careful monitoring of the fetus.

Diabetes controlled by oral hypoglycaemia agents
Oral hypoglycaemic agents are not advised in pregnancy and conversion to the basal insulin regime is best done before conception, if possible. Such women are then monitored in the same way as women with established insulin dependent diabetes.

Gestational diabetes
Gestational diabetes is diagnosed when a woman develops abnormal glucose tolerance for the first time in pregnancy; a small number of such women will remain diabetic after the pregnancy. Currently, many hospitals will perform a random blood glucose test during the antenatal course, interpreting the result in relation to the timing of the last meal. Women with high values will then have a glucose tolerance test or have blood glucose concentrations measured serially (preprandial and postprandial tests three times a day) to determine whether they are glucose intolerant.

Women with gestational diabetes do not have an increased rate of babies with congenital abnormalities but the babies are at risk of being large. There is no consensus on treatment, which ranges from controlling dietary intake to insulin treatment and dietary control. Such women usually have labour induced at term and are at risk of having long labours and babies with shoulder dystocia.

After delivery insulin should be stopped; all affected women should have a glucose tolerance test at six weeks. About 40–60% of such women will develop non-insulin dependent diabetes (type II) in later life but this proportion rises to 70% among those who are obese.

Thyroid disease

Hyperthyroidism
Women who are already hyperthyroid are usually receiving treatment, which may have to be continued throughout pregnancy. The most commonly used drugs are carbimazole and propyl-thiouracil; the former is in more common use but the latter is often chosen in pregnancy as it is less often associated with congenital abnormalities of the scalp. The minimum dose should be prescribed to alleviate any symptoms and to suppress free thyroxine concentration to the normal range. However, some of these women find that their hyperthyroidism ameliorates in the last weeks of pregnancy. In such cases withdrawal of antithyroid drugs may reduce the severity of any fetal goitre.

These women should be tested for the presence of IgG thyroid antibodies (long-acting thyroid stimulator and thyroid receptor antibodies) as these cross the placenta and cause neonatal thyrotoxicosis when present in high titres. Thyroid

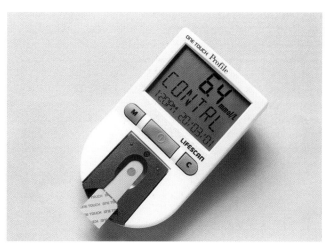

Figure 8.4 Blood glucose concentration meter for home use

Box 8.3   Vaginal delivery in diabetic mothers
- *Good prognostic features*
  - Primigravida <30 years
  - Multigravida with good obstetric history
  - Estimated fetal weight <3500 g
  - Well engaged cephalic presentation
  - Stable diabetic control
- *Bad prognostic features*
  - Primigravida >30 years
  - Multigravida with poor obstetric history
  - Large fetus (>3500 g)
  - Non-engageable head or breech presentation
  - Unstable diabetes

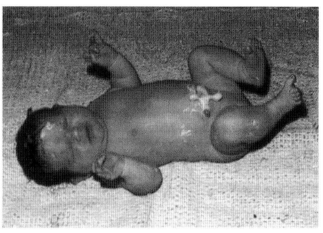

Figure 8.5 A typically large baby born to a diabetic mother

Table 8.2   Effect of thyrotoxicosis and pregnancy on some thyroid tests

	Thyrotoxicosis	Pregnancy
Tri-iodothyronine:		
free	Increased	No change
protein bound	Increased	Increased
Thyroxine:		
free	Increased	No change
protein bound	Increased	Increased
Thyroxine binding		
globulin	No change	Increased

crises (storm crises) are now rare in pregnancy and the immediate puerperium. They are best treated with iodine, which works quicker than β blockade and carbimazole. Operation on the thyroid is rarely indicated in pregnancy but is safest in the middle trimester.

Hypothyroidism

Hypothyroid women are commonly anovular. If they are receiving adequate replacement treatment, however, they ovulate as normal. Such treatment should be continued and may need to be increased during pregnancy.

Epilepsy

An epileptic woman will often consult before becoming pregnant as she may have heard of the potential hazards of antiepileptic drugs. Most antiepileptic drugs have teratogenic properties to a varying extent, but it must be emphasised that epileptic women have an inbuilt increased risk of having babies with malformations even without treatment. This risk should be carefully balanced against the risks to the embryo if the woman has a series of convulsions when anticonvulsant treatment is withdrawn in early pregnancy.

Generally, the woman may stop or modify treatment after full consultation when she has not had a recent fit. However, if the epilepsy is well controlled, there is little point in changing antiepileptics in pregnancy. If she needs treatment the same dose must be continued; phenytoin treatment may be associated with a slightly lower risk of fetal neural tube defects and might be substituted instead of valproate or carbamazepine.

Seizure frequency seems to be the same in pregnancy as outside pregnancy for most epileptic women; if the rate of fitting worsens, blood concentrations of all anticonvulsants should be checked as overdose as well as underdose may be responsible for loss of seizure control.

Prophylactic folic acid (5 mg/day) should be given before and during pregnancy as folate absorption is changed by the antiepileptic drugs. Vitamin K should be given to all the newborn infants of such mothers for similar reasons.

Status epilepticus is unusual in a pregnant woman unless she is known to be a severe epileptic. Diazepam is the best drug to use.

HIV infection

The human immune suppression retrovirus (HIV) attacks CD 4 lymphocytes leading to their suppression and hence increasing susceptibility to infection. The acquired immune deficiency syndrome (AIDS) is the end stage of such a process and develops some years after the initial HIV infection. Transplacental transmission of the virus antenatally from mother to fetus or breast feeding after delivery can lead to an infected baby.

HIV infection is found more commonly in the big towns such as London where 1 in 600 antenatal attenders is HIV positive. In the country generally it is nearer 1 in 10 000. It is probable that pregnancy does not increase the progression of the disease in the mother.

The baby will be infected in 15–20% of cases.[1] There is a possibility that elective caesarean section would reduce this risk by eliminating fetal exposure to the secretions of the genital tract. The European Study, considering 1000 mother/baby pairs, considered that caesarean section halved the risk of infection[1] although subsequent analyses have shown only a

Table 8.3   Therapeutic concentrations of anticonvulsants in blood

	mg/l
Phenytoin	10–12
Phenobarbitone	15–40
Carbamazepine	4–12
Primidone	5–12
Ethosuximide	5–12
Valproate	4–100

Box 8.4   Potential effects of epilepsy on the fetus

- Increased risk of epilepsy in the baby:
  - if mother alone affected 4%
  - if both parents affected 15%
  - if another child affected 10%
- Increased risk of congenital abnormalities:
  - if either parent affected
  - if mother takes more than one anti-epileptic drug
- Isolated maternal fits do not usually affect fetus. Status epilepticus does

For most epileptic women the frequency of seizures is not affected by pregnancy.

Box 8.5   Transmission of HIV

Transmission of HIV from mother to fetus may be:

- across the placenta in pregnancy
- due to exposure to blood during vaginal delivery
- by breast feeding

The most frequent cause is vaginal transmission which can be reduced by bypassing the vagina (i.e. CS)

20% reduction due to caesarean section.[2] At present the best prospect of management is to prevent women becoming HIV infected. In pregnancy, the established infected women should be detected by antenatal screening for HIV with proper counselling and offered treatment with anti-retroviral agents, the current product being zidovudine.

It is worth diagnosing HIV in pregnancy for now there is a reasonable treatment which reduces the rate of transmission of HIV to the fetus from 25% in a control group compared with 7% in a zidovudine group.

All infants of HIV positive mothers should be commenced on zidovudine for six weeks and tested at one month and four months for antibodies. Breast feeding is contraindicated in the UK but may be the only method of contraception available in developing countries; the extra risks of HIV transmission should be weighed against further unwanted pregnancies. Folate supplements are especially recommended for the prepregnancy period and the first trimester for all women with HIV infection, to prevent neural tube defects. Infected women who have a high viral load or who have not had any antenatal treatment may be better delivered by caesarean section to reduce the transmission to infants.

Jaundice

The commonest causes of jaundice in pregnancy are the various forms of hepatitis and drugs that affect the liver. Gall stones and severe pre-eclampsia may be responsible, but in the UK gall stones are rare in the age group concerned. Cholestasis in the last trimester may occur spontaneously or follow the use of steroids; fatty degeneration of the liver in the last weeks of pregnancy is very rare but can lead to liver failure as can severe autoimmune disease.

The results of the conventional liver function tests are not as helpful during pregnancy, and the early participation of liver experts in the care of a woman with jaundice during pregnancy is essential.

Anaemia

In pregnancy, anaemia might be due to:

● lack of haemoglobin from a low intake of iron (microcytic anaemia) or of folate (megaloblastic anaemia)
● haemorrhagic anaemia following chronic blood loss
● haemolytic anaemia in those with abnormalities of the genes of the haemoglobin molecule or of the envelope of the red cell.

Iron deficiency anaemia
This is the most common form of anaemia in the UK. The daily need for iron rises from 2 mg per day to 4 mg in pregnancy. This can be provided by improved diet or more practically by taking regular prophylactic tablets containing 60 mg per day of elemental iron. This supplement is given to most pregnant women in the UK. If they cannot take iron tablets, a liquid preparation or intramuscular iron should be provided.

Folate deficiency anaemia
This is less common than iron deficiency anaemia in the UK. Folate needs are increased because of increased maternal demands from growth of the uterus and breasts as well as the increased tissues laid down in the growing fetus.

The woman may produce symptoms of anaemia with breathlessness and pallor; the blood film may show a low

---

Box 8.6   Some causes of jaundice in pregnancy

● *Pregnancy associated*
  • Cholestasis
  • Acute fatty liver of pregnancy
  • Disseminated intravascular coagulopathy
  • Severe pre-eclampsia and HELLP syndrome
  • Excessive vomiting (hyperemesis)
  • Severe septicaemia in late pregnancy

● *Unrelated to pregnancy*
  • Viral hepatitis
  • Drugs
      chlorpromazine
      tetracycline
      steroids
  • Chronic liver disease
  • Gall stones
  • Chronic haemolysis

Table 8.4   Normal haematological values in pregnancy

	Range
Total blood volume (ml)	4000–6000
Red cell volume (ml)	1500–1800
Red cell count (10^{12}/l)	4–5
White cell count (10^9/l)	10–15
Haemoglobin (g/dl)	11.0–13.5
Erythrocyte sedimentation rate (mm/hr)	10–60
Mean corpuscular volume (μm^3)	80–95
Mean corpuscular haemoglobin (pg)	27–32
Serum iron ($\mu mol/l$)	11–25
Total iron binding capacity ($\mu mol/l$)	40–70
Serum ferritin ($\mu g/l$)	10–200
Serum folate ($\mu g/l$)	6–9

Box 8.7   Indices of iron deficiency anaemia

● *Blood film: red cells*
  • normal size or microcytic
  • hypochromic
  • anisocytosis
  • poikilocytosis
● *Haematological values*
  • haemolobin ↓
  • mean corpuscular volume ↓
  • mean corpuscular haemoglobin ↓
  • serum iron ↓
  • serum ferritin ↓

haemoglobin concentration, maybe with macrocytes. The latter may be missing and a bone marrow sample from the iliac crest may be required to show megaloblastic changes.

The condition is treated by oral folate; the diet can be improved and should contain dark green leaf vegetables and yeast extracts. However, in Britain, usually folate is given prophylactically, often combined with iron, to prevent folate deficiency. Those with twins and women taking antibiotics require extra folate. These needs are in addition to the folate used before pregnancy and in early gestation to prevent the formation of central nervous system abnormalities.

Haemorrhagic anaemia

Haemorrhagic anaemia is rare in the UK among women of childbearing age, but chronic bleeding from peptic ulceration, aspirin ingestion, or piles may occur. In other countries tapeworms or hookworms may cause a constant chronic blood loss. Treatment is that of the causative condition.

Haemolytic anaemia

Hereditary haemolytic anaemia is also a rare disease in the white population of the United Kingdom, but other races may show a variety of haemolytic anaemias.

Haemoglobinopathies

Women liable to haemoglobinopathies and their antecedents usually come from Mediterranean countries or Asia and are often known to the family doctor beforehand. All such women should have a blood film examined and their blood checked by electrophoresis at the booking clinic. If they are found to be carriers, their partner's blood should be checked. If they too are carriers, fetal diagnosis is available from early chorionic villus sampling and from fetal blood sampling in later pregnancy. Such women are best managed at special combined antenatal-haematological units and should be sent to such hospitals early in pregnancy so that plans can be made to cover all eventualities. If not, as luck would have it, the crisis will always come on Saturday night at 11.30 pm.

Sickle cell disease

Most women in the UK have haemoglobin A. Defective genes can alter the amino acid sequence of haemoglobin, which may produce symptoms. Haemoglobin S originated in the Middle East but is now found in Africa and the West Indies. Those with haemoglobin C come from West Africa. The partner's blood should be tested and antenatal diagnosis of the fetus is available by direct gene probe from a chorionic villus sample if both partners carry the trait.

In pregnancy a woman with sickle cell disease is at high risk of complications; she deserves special antenatal supervision. Even in experienced hands the perinatal mortality rate can be four times that in a normal population and maternal mortality is also greatly increased. In extreme cases sickling produces crises, leading to sudden pain in the bones, chest, or abdomen after small vessel infarction. Rates of severe pre-eclampsia are higher, as are the incidences of chest and urinary infections. Intrauterine growth retardation and fetal death occur because of placental infarction.

If a crisis occurs then both haemoglobin concentration and red cell volume should be checked every few hours. Hospital treatment with intravenous hydration, partial exchange transfusion or packed red cell transfusions, and antibiotics may be required. Women with haemoglobin concentrations below 6.0 g/dl should have exchange transfusions before elective

Table 8.5 Dose and ferrous iron content of commonly prescribed iron tablets

Iron tablets	Dose (mg)	Ferrous iron content (mg)
Ferrous sulphate (dried)	200	60
Ferrous sulphate	300	60
Ferrous fumarate	200	65
Ferrous gluconate	300	35
Ferrous succinate	100	35

Box 8.8 Indices of folate deficiency anaemia

- *Blood film*
  - red cells
    - normal size or macrocytic
    - normochromic
    - anisocytosis
    - poikilocytosis
    - sometimes nuclear material
  - white cells
    - leucopenia
    - hypersegmentation
  - platelets
    - sometimes thrombocytopenia
- *Haematological values*
  - haemoglobin ↓
  - mean corpuscular volume ↓ or =
  - mean corpuscular haemoglobin ↑
  - serum iron ↑
  - red cell folate ↓
  - marrow megaloblastosis

Box 8.9 Indices of sickle cell anaemia

- *Blood film*
  - red cells
    - polychromasia
    - sickle cells
    - Howell-Jolly bodies
  - white cells
    - leucocytosis
  - platelets
    - thrombocytosis
- *Check*
  - haemoglobin electrophoresis
  - test partner

Box 8.10 Treatment of sickle cell crisis

- Pethidine for pain
- Antibiotic only if infection also
- Oxygen
- Intravenous fluids to maintain hydration
- ? Intravenous bicarbonates for acidaemia
- ? Exchange transfusion

delivery. Babies of high risk couples should be tested and followed up if they have sickle cell disease.

Thalassaemia

In thalassaemia, the life of a red cell is shorter than the usual 120 days and so anaemia follows because there is a more rapid breakdown than production of cells. Haemoglobin concentration is low but the serum iron concentration is high.

Again, iron may not be needed if stores are adequate but many such women need extra iron as iron deficiency anaemia may accompany thalassaemia. The stress of hypoxia or acidaemia should be avoided as both increase the breakdown rate of red cells.

Urinary tract infection

Acute urinary infection occurs in about 2% of women during pregnancy. Infection of the urethra and trigone of the bladder is signalled by dysuria and increased frequency of micturition, whereas infection of the upper tract affecting the ureters or kidney produces loin pain and spikes of fever.

A midstream urine specimen should be checked for the presence of cells and bacteria (with bacterial sensitivity to antibiotics) before any treatment is started. The woman should drink much more and take a wide spectrum antibiotic such as amoxycillin until the results of the test are known. Antibiotic treatment may have to be changed according to the sensitivity results but usually amoxycillin suffices. (Alkalination of the urine may be performed, though this is unpleasant and entails taking potassium citrate mixture.)

After 7–10 days, a second midstream specimen of urine should be sent to the laboratory. If bacteria are still detected, continuous low dose antibotic prophylaxis using trimethoprim (second and third trimesters only) or amoxycillin should be considered. Cranberry juice may be useful in preventing recurrent infection.

Asymptomatic bacteriuria

Infection may be low grade and asymptomatic. About 4% of pregnant women have evidence of bacterial infection of the urine; its significance level is arbitrarily set at more than 100 000 bacteria per ml of urine.

If all women are screened early in pregnancy and asymptomatic bacteriuria is detected it is probably wise to treat, as the risk of developing acute pyelonephritis in pregnancy is about 30%. Treatment is for five days with an antibiotic to which the bacteria are sensitive. A urine sample should be recultured 14 days later. If bacteria are still present continuous antibiotic prophylaxis should be considered.

Any woman with persistent asymptomatic bacteriuria through pregnancy should have her urinary tract checked after delivery. About 20% of this subgroup will be found to have a structural abnormality of the kidneys, ureters, or bladder.

Chronic renal disease

Most women with chronic renal disease are well known to their general practitioner and have usually been counselled by a renal physician about the risks of pregnancy and the precautions required. In brief, renal function usually improves in pregnancy, and there is no evidence that pregnancy adversely affects the long-term prognosis from the renal disease. The outlook in pregnancy is favourable if the patient is not hypertensive and does not have proteinuria before pregnancy. Pregnancy should be carefully supervised by the obstetric and renal team.

Box 8.11   Indices of thalassaemia

- *Blood film*
  - red cells
    - ? polychromasia
    - microcytosis
    - hypochromia
    - sometimes anisocytosis
    - sometimes poikilocytosis
    - target cells present
- *Haematological values*
  - haemoglobin ↓
  - serum iron ↓
  - mean corpuscular volume ↓
  - mean corpuscular haemoglobin ↓
- *Check*
  - haemoglobin electrophoresis
  - test partner

Box 8.12   Acute urinary infection in pregnancy

- Check MSSU for organisms and sensitivity
- Use as first line drug
  - amoxycillin or
  - ampicillin or
  - cephalosporin or
  - augmentin
- Be prepared to change if sensitivity tests indicate
- Use with caution if sensitivity demands
  - sulphonamides (beware kernicterus in baby)
  - trimethoprim (beware of folic acid antagonism)
  - nitrofurantoin (because of G6PD deficiency in baby)

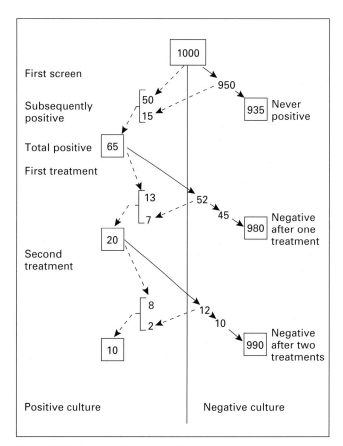

Figure 8.6 Progress of 1000 women with asymptomatic bacteriuria during pregnancy

Transplant recipients have normal fertility. There is little evidence that the commonly used immunosuppressive agents cause an excess of fetal abnormalities. Episodes of rejection are not more common in childbirth, but if they occur they usually do so in the puerperium. If the transplanted kidney is in the pelvis a caesarean section may be necessary for mechanical reasons.

Abdominal pain in early pregnancy

From the uterus
Miscarriage
One of the commonest causes of pain in early pregnancy is spontaneous miscarriage. This subject is dealt with in Chapter 7.

Retroverted uterus
Retroversion is a common position for a normal uterus. In pregnancy the uterus expands into the abdomen. If adhesions are present, however, this cannot occur; by 10–12 weeks the enlarging uterus fills the pelvis and pain is associated with retention of urine. The urethra is stretched by the uterine bulk and the bladder pushed to the abdomen so that urine cannot pass. These findings can be confirmed by ultrasonography.

Management includes draining the urine with an indwelling catheter. The cure eventually comes when the uterus grows into the general abdominal cavity by anterior sacculation, so relieving the urethral stretch.

Fibroids
Fibroids are found in older pregnant women (those aged 30–40), particularly among Afro-Caribbean women. In pregnancy fibroids can undergo torsion if they are subserous; this is more common in the puerperium. Red degeneration is commonest at 12–18 weeks of pregnancy but can occur throughout, with resulting necrobiosis in the fibroid. The woman presents with tenderness over the mass accompanied by vomiting and mild fever.

Red degeneration is self limiting; if the diagnosis is firm, management is bedrest with analgesia and intravenous correction of any dehydration. Ultrasound may help to confirm the presence of fibroids, although necrobiosis may not show clearly. In truly doubtful cases, as in a low-right sided fibroid that mimics appendicitis, a laparotomy should be performed to exclude surgically correctable conditions. If red degeneration is diagnosed the surgeon would do well not to remove the fibroid at this stage but to close the abdomen and continue conservative management.

From the fallopian tube
Ectopic pregnancy
Unruptured ectopic pregnancy causes chronic symptoms and needs to be managed in hospital whereas ruptured ectopic pregnancy produces acute symptoms and collapse and needs urgent hospital management. The condition is dealt with in Chapter 7.

Torsion
Torsion is uncommon and occurs mainly in younger women during early pregnancy when a long tube may twist on its pedicle accompanied by torsion of the ovary, especially if the latter has a cyst in it.

The woman has non-specific hypogastric pain and a constant area of tenderness suprapubically on the lateral edge

Box 8.13 Considerations for pregnancy in chronic renal disease
- Type of disease
  - beware scleroderma, periarteritis nodosa
- Blood pressure
  - diastolic pressure <90 mm Hg
- Renal function
  - plasma creatinine <250 µmol/l
  - plasma urea <10 mmol/l
  - no proteinuria
- Review essential drug treatment

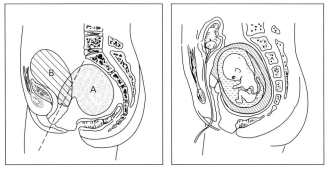
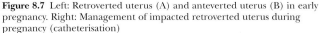

Figure 8.7 Left: Retroverted uterus (A) and anteverted uterus (B) in early pregnancy. Right: Management of impacted retroverted uterus during pregnancy (catheterisation)

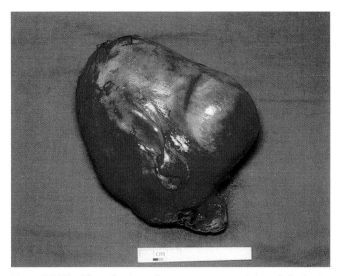

Figure 8.8 Fibroids are benign quiescent tumours consisting of whorls of fibres and few cells

If you do not think of an ectopic pregnancy you will not diagnose one. Always consider unruptured ectopic pregnancy in any young woman having sexual intercourse who has lower abdominal pain.

Box 8.14 Fibroids in pregnancy
- Usually increase in size but become hypovascular
- Necrobiosis (red degeneration) is painful but treat conservatively
- Torsion of subserous fibroid is acutely painful and needs surgical removal

of the rectus abdominis muscle. Ultrasound does not help but diagnostic laparoscopy in early pregnancy is useful. A laparotomy is required; if the lateral end of the fallopian tube is non-viable it must be resected; in rare cases the ovary is also ischaemic and requires removal.

From the pelvic ligaments
Round ligament
These stretch as the uterus rises in the abdomen and pulls on the uterine round ligaments like an inflating hot air balloon tugging its guyropes. Usually the ligaments stretch easily, but if the pull is too strong small haematomas occur. This commonly starts at 16–20 weeks' gestation.

On examination tenderness is localized over the round ligament and often radiates down to the pubic tubercle alongside the symphysis pubis.

Treatment is bedrest, analgesia, and local warmth.

From the ovary
Ovarian tumours
In early pregnancy an ovarian cystic tumour may rupture to release the contents of the cyst, irritating the parietal peritoneum. Bleeding may occur into a corpus luteal cyst. An ultrasound scan may confirm the diagnosis, and a laparotomy is indicated if the clinical situation does not settle. At laparotomy, only that part of the ovary containing the cyst should be removed. If it is a luteal cyst, conservation is necessary as the corpus luteum is probably the major source of progesterone in the first trimester and some of this metabolism continues into later gestation.

Extrapelvic causes
Vomiting
Though many women who vomit in pregnancy have little upset, vomiting or retching may be sufficiently severe to cause muscle ache from stretch. The upper abdominal wall is tender and no specific masses can be felt. If a woman is vomiting this much it is probably wise to admit her to hospital for intravenous fluids, antiemetic treatment, and sedation to allow her intestinal tract some peace. The pain usually settles down as the vomiting decreases.

Pyelonephritis
Stasis in the urinary tract associated with ascending urinary infection often follows dilatation of the ureters (due to raised progesterone concentrations) and the pressure of the increasing uterus on the bladder. It is most likely in mid-pregnancy, when the woman presents with vomiting, symptoms of fever, and low hypogastric or loin pain.

Appendicitis
Appendicitis and pregnancy both occur in young women and therefore may occur concurrently by chance. The incidence of appendicitis in pregnancy is not increased but its diagnosis may be more difficult. For this reason and because of a reluctance to operate, appendicitis used to have a high mortality and morbidity in pregnancy.

As it grows, the uterus displaces the caecum from the right iliac fossa upwards and sideways, so the inflamed appendix may present with symptoms and signs in unexpected places. No longer tucked into the right iliac fossa, the appendix is now in the general abdomen and is less easy to wall off by omentum and gut when it becomes inflamed; generalized peritonitis is commoner in pregnant than non-pregnant women.

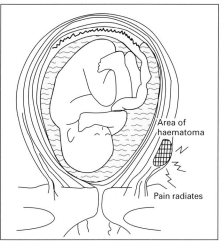

Figure 8.9 Haematoma of round ligament

Box 8.15   Ovarian pain in pregnancy
- Tortion of pedicle of ovary with lateral end of tube
- Stretch of capsule of a cyst
- Bleeding into cavity of cyst (corpus luteum)
- Rupture of cyst with release of contents

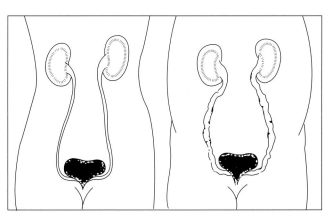

Figure 8.10 During pregnancy the ureters lengthen and become more tortuous and dilated

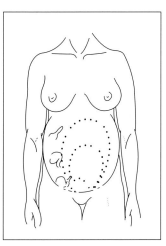

Figure 8.11 The site of the appendix changes as pregnancy advances

A history may elicit the characteristic pain shift, although it is not always localised to the right iliac fossa. Nausea and anorexia occur, sometimes confused by the symptoms of pregnancy. The tenderness over the appendix will shift higher as pregnancy continues. The treatment is operation, the incision being placed over the point of maximum tenderness marked by the surgeon before anaesthesia. Occasionally the results of a rectal examination can be falsely reassuring if the appendix has migrated from the area reached by an examining finger.

The previous reluctance to operate must be overcome; anyone suspected of having appendicitis in pregnancy should have a laparotomy by an experienced surgeon. Even in late pregnancy, caesarean section is not necessary at the same time unless the woman is in labour; women can have a normal vaginal delivery within a few days of an appendicectomy.

Other causes

Cholecystitis is commoner among women who live in or originate from countries whose residents characteristically have high cholesterol diets such as Australia and New Zealand. The pain is usually upper right abdominal with tenderness centred on the eighth or ninth rib tip. Treatment in the absence of jaundice is conservative with antibiotics or removal, depending on the surgical need.

Volvulus of large bowel can occur in pregnancy, though it presents more characteristically in the puerperium.

Small bowel colic may follow an attack of gastroenteritis. *Urinary lithiasis* occurs in the same frequency in pregnancy as in non-pregnant women.

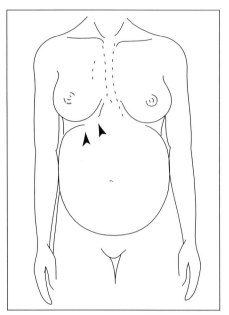

Figure 8.12 Pain in cholecystitis

Abdominal pain in late pregnancy

From the uterus

Uterine contractions

All pregnancies end in labour, which may occur well before term. Premature labour can present with abdominal pain, taking the woman and sometimes her general practitioner by surprise. Usually the pain is intermittent and recurrent and the uterus can be felt contracting coincidentally with the pain. There may be a loss of mucus or a little blood from the vagina, on vaginal examination the cervix is soft, thin, taken up, and sometimes dilated. When labour is very preterm (26–32 weeks) the woman should be transferred to a hospital with an expert neonatal unit rather than necessarily to the one where she has booked (see Chapter 12).

Placental abruption

Separation of the placenta from its bed before the third stage of labour is painful and results in shock (see Chapter 10).

Extraperitoneal causes

Pregnancy-induced hypertension

In severe fulminating pregnancy-induced hypertension a woman may complain of epigastric pain associated with vomiting. She will probably have raised blood pressure and proteinuria with oedema and be known to be hypertensive. There may also be visual symptoms (outlined in Chapter 9).

Rectus haematoma

Very rarely the rectus muscle may dehisce and the inferior epigastric veins behind the muscle rupture. As the anterior

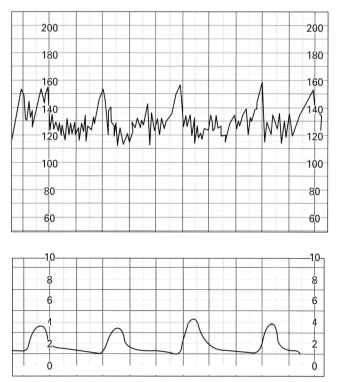

Figure 8.13 A cardiotocograph in early labour showing the fetal heart rate (above) and the regular uterine contractions every three minutes (below)

abdominal wall is greatly overstretched by the uterus, a fit of sneezing could cause this. Pain is severe and usually localised to one segment of the muscle. Blood loss is slight with the haematoma but increases if the veins rupture. Rectus haematoma is diagnosed from the fact that pain and tenderness worsen when the woman contracts the rectus muscles by raising her head. Ultrasound is helpful.

If the diagnosis is firm, management is conservative, but in doubtful cases a laparotomy should be performed, and haematoma behind the rectus muscle confirms the diagnosis.

Pelvic arthropathy

Relaxation of the ligaments guarding the pelvic joints follows the secretion of the hormone relaxin. This allows appreciable separation of the symphysis pubis, giving abdominal pain that is much aggravated by walking. In extreme cases weight bearing is impossible and the woman has to retire to bed completely. Treatment is rest; binders are of little help. Vaginal delivery should be anticipated. This condition may take up to two months to resolve after delivery, but it usually does slowly get better. Severe cases may last for up to a year, and long-term follow-up is wise.

Conclusion

Most women who present with abdominal pain in pregnancy may have nothing serious the matter. Pain can, however, lead the doctor to diagnose a serious condition, when action needs to be taken. As investigations play a small part in many of these diagnoses, experienced general practitioners can often diagnose its cause and continue the management of many women at home, but if there is any doubt the local obstetric department ought to be consulted.

> All general medical conditions are modified by pregnancy; diagnosis may be clouded and treatment may have to be changed. Early abdominal examination will usually help differentiate serious from lesser conditions. If the condition is thought to be serious consult an obstetrician early rather than send to a general surgeon.

References

1 European Collaborative Study. Caesarian section and the risk of vertical transmission of HIV-1 infection. *Lancet* 1994;**343**:1464–7.
2 Dunn D, Newell M, Mayaux M *et al*. Mode of delivery and vertical transmission of HIV-1. *J AIDS* 1994;**7**:1064–6.

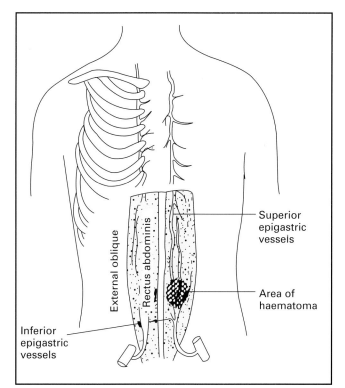

Figure 8.14 A rectus haematoma usually arises from the inferior epigastric vessels deep in the rectus muscle

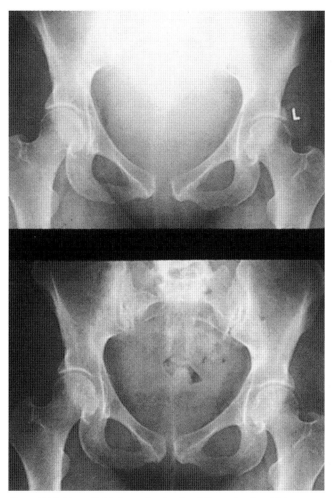

Figure 8.15 Above: Pelvis immediately after delivery showing dehiscence of pubic symphysis. Below: Same pelvis six weeks later. Imaging by ultrasonography reduces the risks of irradiation in a young woman

Recommended reading

- Johnstone F. *HIV and pregnancy.* Year of Obstetrics and Gynaecology, Volume 8. London: RCOG Press, 2000.
- Nelson-Piercy C. *A handbook of obstetric medicine.* Oxford: Isis Medical Media, 2000.
- Rubin P. *Prescribing in pregnancy,* 2nd edn. London: BMJ Publishing Group, 1995.
- Sbarouni E, Oakley C. Outcome of pregnancy in women with valve prosthesis. *Br Heart J* 1994; **71**:176–201.

The table showing therapeutic concentration of anticonvulsants is based on that by J Donaldson in *Critical care of the obstetric patient,* edited by R Berkowitz, and is reproduced by permission of Churchill Livingstone. The photographs of the glucose testing equipment are reproduced by permission of Boehringer Mannheim (United Kingdom).

9 Raised blood pressure in pregnancy

One of the original aims of promaternity (antenatal) care in 1901 was the prevention of fits and convulsions due to eclampsia, which was often associated with pre-eclampsia. The term pre-eclampsia has been refined in later years as eclampsia now occurs rarely.

Raised blood pressure affects the fetus as well as the mother. In the later weeks of pregnancy it may fall into one of several categories.

- Chronic hypertension is present before the 20th week and has causes outside pregnancy.
- Pregnancy-induced hypertension develops after the 20th week of pregnancy and usually resolves within 10 days of delivery.
- Pregnancy-induced hypertension with proteinuria now is called pre-eclampsia and occurs mostly in primigravidas.
- Pregnancy-induced hypertension with or without proteinuria may be superimposed on chronic hypertension and this is a most dangerous combination, the effects of pregnancy being added to those of chronic hypertension.
- Eclampsia is a convulsive condition usually associated with proteinuric hypertension.

Causes

The mechanism of pregnancy-induced hypertension is now almost completely understood, with reasonable educated guesses being possible in unknown cases. The primary defect is failure of the second wave of trophoblastic invasion into the decidua. Usually the trophoblast invades the entire length of the spiral arteries by 22 weeks of gestation. This leads to an appreciable fall in peripheral resistance and therefore a fall in blood pressure. In addition, as the trophoblast usually removes all the muscle coat of the spiral arteries, blood flows unimpeded into the intervillous space, gushing like a fountain over the villous tree that contains the fetal vessels. This ensures adequate time for exchange of oxygen, nutrients, and the waste products of metabolism.

If the second wave of trophoblastic invasion fails, the peripheral resistance does not fall and the haemodynamic mechanisms are not reset for the increased vascular space of pregnancy. Furthermore, the muscle coats retained by the spiral arterioles are sensitive to circulating pressor agents, particularly angiotension II. Most of the hypertensive changes are due to hormonal rather than sympathetic nervous system influence. At the spiral arterioles, the reduced volume of trophoblast leads to an imbalance in the prostacyclin–thromboxane system. The comparative overproduction of thromboxane encourages vasospasm of the spiral arteries and also local platelet aggregation. The lower concentrations of prostacyclin remove the protection that pregnancy offers against angiotension II.

The damaged muscle coating and intima of the spiral arteries undergoes acute atherosis, an accelerated form of arteriosclerosis that further narrows and then occludes the arterioles. A further increase in blood pressure follows, and the decrease in perfusion of the intervillous space leads commonly to intrauterine growth retardation.

Low dose aspirin may reduce the severity of pregnancy-induced hypertension in patients at risk, moderating the disease once established. The mode of action is irreversible

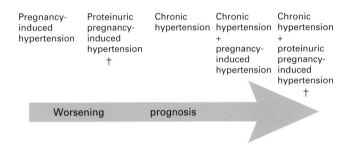

Box 9.1   Some accepted definitions of raised blood pressure

- Hypertension
  - Mild—diastolic blood pressure >90 mm Hg
  - Severe—diastolic blood pressure >110 mm Hg

- Pregnancy-induced hypertension
  - Mild—diastolic blood pressure >90 mm Hg after the 20th week of pregnancy with no raised blood pressure beforehand and no proteinuria
  - Moderate—diastolic blood pressure >100 mm Hg after the 20th week of pregnancy with no raised blood pressure beforehand and no proteinuria
  - Severe—diastolic blood pressure >90 mm Hg after the 20th week of pregnancy with no raised blood pressure beforehand but with any degree of proteinuria

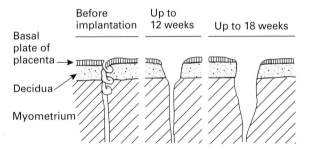

Figure 9.1 Permutations of hypertensive disease in pregnant and non-pregnant women. †These are designated as pre-eclampsia

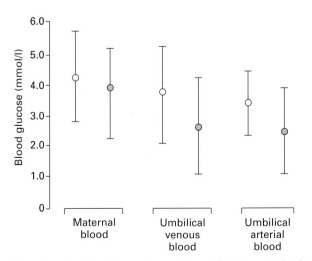

Figure 9.2 The invasion of spiral arteries by the trophoblast converts them into deltas and so improves blood flow

Figure 9.3 Transfer of glucose from mother to fetus in babies who show normal growth (○) and in those who are small for gestational age

poisoning of platelet cyclo-oxygenase. This probably prevents or delays clotting in the spiral arterioles.

The effects of pregnancy-induced hypertension on organs other than the placenta are mediated by the effects of hypertension or by activation of the complement system. This causes immune complexes to be deposited on the basement membrane of the kidney and allows protein to leak into the urine. In severe disease platelets are both consumed and activated so that coagulopathy may follow.

Management

Though pregnancy-induced hypertension develops out of the blue, particularly in first pregnancies, many women who already have hypertension will wonder about becoming pregnant and the effects that the pregnancy may have on their underlying hypertension. This matter should be considered carefully before a woman becomes pregnant, and if necessary the woman should be referred to a local prepregnancy advisory service. Since tobacco is associated with increased risks of cardiovascular disease in general, one would expect smoking mothers to have a higher rate of pre-eclampsia. This is not so and many studies have shown that smoking is associated with lower rates of pre-eclampsia. However, if it does occur it is often more severe in the smoker.

Generally speaking, if the blood pressure is not very high, or it can be kept low with antihypertensive drugs, and if there is no concomitant proteinuria before pregnancy, most women will have a successful pregnancy. They should continue their antihypertensive treatment in pregnancy.

Women with renal damage already leading to proteinuria and those who have diastolic pressures above 100 mm Hg despite adequate antihypertensive treatment should be investigated more thoroughly. Such women have a three to seven times increased risk above background of developing pregnancy-induced hypertension on top of their disease and the prognosis is worse for both mother and baby.

The ideal start to the management of pregnancy-induced hypertension, with or without proteinuria, is to detect it early. Each visit to the antenatal clinic includes a blood pressure recording. Recently, women likely to develop pregnancy-induced hypertension have been detected before this happens at 24 weeks by the use of Doppler measurements of blood flow velocity of uterine arteries, from which a measure of placental vascular resistance is derived. Doppler investigation may become available as a screening test in the next few years, providing, for example, an indicator of which women would benefit from low dose aspirin. Once prostaglandin was shown to be involved, an obvious antidote seemed to be aspirin and for a while this was in favour. Unfortunately the randomised CLASP study showed that in 9264 women there was only a 12% reduction in the incidence of proteinuria pre-eclampsia which was not significant.[1] Another possible organic cause of proteinuric hypertension has been the reduction of nitric oxide. This has led to the use of glyceryl trinitrate patches but this is still in the realms of research.

Once raised blood pressure is established, rest is usually central to primary management. Without accompanying proteinuria, the woman may be treated at home, where rest must take priority over everything else, including work at home or outside and care of other members of the family. Those with other children find it difficult to follow this regime and probably a third of women do not rest when so advised. If the hypertension increases despite proper bedrest, or proteinuria follows, admission to hospital is required.

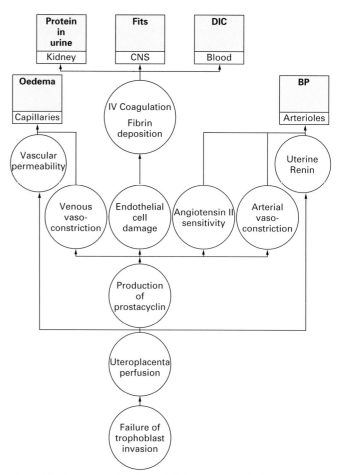

Figure 9.4 The suggested pathways (–O–) of pregnancy-induced hypertension changes related to their outcomes (☐)

Table 9.1 Risk factors for the development of pregnancy-induced hypertension

Risk factors	Ratio
Nulliparity	3:1
Age above 40 years	3:1
Chronic hypertension	10:1
Chronic renal disease	20:1
Twins	2:1

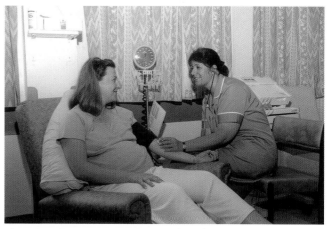

Figure 9.5 Blood pressure measurement is a simple and useful screening test when performed repeatedly by standardised techniques. All doctors and midwives in a unit should use the same criterion for diastolic pressure—probably the loss of phase V Korotkoff sound

In hospital rest will be reinforced and the condition will be monitored by using ultrasound measurements of the growth of the fetus, Doppler measurements of blood velocity in the umbilical arteries and some would measure flow in the uterine arteries. Cardiotocographic measurements of variations in the fetal heart rate may also be used. Plasma urate concentrations and an increase in the liver enzyme aspartate transferase are useful biochemical indicators of deterioration, and a fall in the platelet count reflects severe disease. (The HELLP Syndrome – Haemolgia Elevated Liver Enzymes, Low Platelets). The management of severe hypertension now no longer includes treatment with sedatives or diuretics; sedatives tend merely to reduce the mother's level of consciousness and cross the placenta, causing depression of the fetal central and peripheral nervous systems. Similarly, diuretics are of little use, except for the relief of acutely painful oedema. They may even be harmful by reducing plasma volume and therefore perfusion of the placental bed.

Antihypertensive drugs are useful in protecting the mother's circulation, mostly against the risk of a stroke. They have no effect on the progression of the pregnancy-induced hypertension or on fetal growth but they help to maintain the pregnancy longer, so allowing the fetus to become more mature. These drugs tend to be kept for women whose hypertension increases despite bedrest. Methyldopa is still the commonest oral drug used in the short term. Hydralazine is given intravenously as first aid in acutely deteriorating hypertension. Combined α and β blockers, such as labetalol, are gaining in popularity because they give better control.

Calcium channel blockers such as nifedipine are being used more widely for they are effective in the control of acute hypertension. No serious fetal side effects occur although maternal side effects of flushing and headache may demand discontinuation.

The final and ultimate treatment of pregnancy-induced hypertension is delivery. Induction of labour or caesarean section should be reserved until the fetus is mature enough for the neonatal facilities available, but it must be used when the condition deteriorates. Two changes in managing pregnancy-induced hypertension have considerably altered the outlook for mother and fetus.

- Firstly, use of antihypertensive drugs to allow the fetus to spend longer in the uterus has spread rapidly and widely. Formerly, such drugs were thought to reduce placental bed perfusion and so affect the fetus deleteriously; their use in pregnancy was restricted. Now most obstetricians use them, and by reducing maternal risk, pregnancy is prolonged by a few more weeks so that the child is more mature.
- Secondly, the obstetrician's reluctance to perform a caesarean section earlier in pregnancy has diminished. With improved intensive neonatal care, caesarean section as early as 28 weeks gives a reasonable chance of fetal survival. The worst effects of prolonged renal and cerebral damage are reduced for the mother and the fetus is delivered before being affected by serious chronic hypoxia *in utero*.

The treatment of women with severe pregnancy-induced hypertension is best performed in special regional hypertension units, where neonatal and obstetric care is planned together. The Confidential Enquiries into Maternal Deaths have urged for years that each Health Authority should have one or more such designated units. A woman with or at risk of severe pregnancy-induced hypertension should be admitted to such a unit to obtain the best concentrated and coordinated obstetric and neonatal care.

The future management of pregnancy-induced hypertension may lie in the reduction of platelet agglutination during early

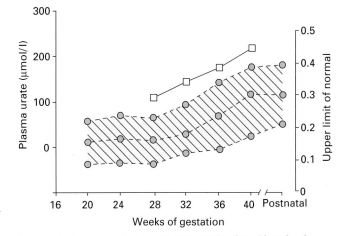

Figure 9.6 Changes in plasma urate concentration from 16 weeks of gestation showing 10th, 50th, and 90th centiles and the accepted upper limit of normal values. ❑—❑ shows the levels in a woman with severe pre-eclampsia

Table 9.2 Drugs and dosages used in treatment of pregnancy-induced hypertension

Drug	Route	Dosage	Comment
Centrally acting drugs			
Clonidine	Oral	500–100 µg three times a day	
Methyldopa	Oral	250–1000 mg daily	Safe to use
Vasodilators			
Sodium nitroprusside	Intravenous	0.3–1.0 µg/kg/min	Only for short-term use
Hydralazine	Intravenous	5–20 mg over 20 minutes	Drug of choice in emergency
β Adrenoceptor blockers			
Propranolol	Oral	80–160 mg daily	Used to be thought to reduce placental perfusion
α and β Adrenoceptor blockers			
Labetalol	Intravenous	50 mg over a minute	Water soluble and so crosses placenta; may not be effective in acute problem
	Oral	100–200 mg daily	

The ultimate treatment of pregnancy-induced hypertension is delivery.

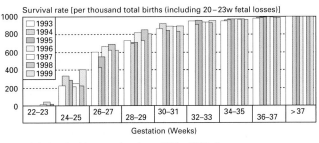

Figure 9.7 Survival by gestational age, Wales 1993–9

pregnancy, so preventing damage to the placental bed. This might halt the whole cascade of problems. Aspirin in early pregnancy might block the cyclo-oxygenase enzymes of the platelets so that they would not be able to produce thromboxane. It was thought that low dose aspirin (75 mg a day) may be helpful in mitigating the worst effects of pregnancy-induced hypertension with proteinuria but the published results of the CLASP study do not substantiate this.[1]

Eclampsia

Imminent eclampsia

The old term fulminating pre-eclampsia is less often used, but semantics are not as important as the recognition of this severe, acute change in a woman's condition. Having had moderate or even severe but symptom-free pregnancy-induced hypertension with proteinuria, the woman suddenly starts to produce symptoms. She may have frontal headaches and visual symptoms with jagged, angular flashes at the periphery of her visual fields and loss of vision in areas, both symptoms being due to cerebral oedema. She often has epigastric pain due to stretch of the peritoneum over the oedematous liver. In addition, some women have a curious itch confined to the mask region of the face. On examination her blood pressure may be much raised above previous readings or proteinuria may increase sharply; she may have increased and brisk reflex responses at knee and clonus. This woman needs urgent hypotensive and anticonvulsant treatment. If she is at home she should be admitted, with intravenous diazepam and, if necessary, hydralazine running continuously. Diazepam prevents fits and hydralazine reduces blood pressure but magnesium sulphate does both.[2]

Eclampsia

Convulsions associated with pregnancy-induced hypertension are termed eclampsia; they are very similar in form to those of epilepsy. Occasionally women in the beginning of the third trimester have eclamptic fits, having had perfectly normal blood pressure readings and urine test results within the previous few weeks at the routine visits to the antenatal clinic. Most women with eclampsia, however, give prodromal signs of pregnancy-induced hypertension with proteinuria in pregnancy; most are preterm (<37 weeks) while a fifth are before 32 weeks. The fits may develop in labour or the puerperium, the first day after birth having the highest risk.

The general practitioner's first move is to control the fits and prevent them causing damage to the woman. She should be laid on her side and an airway established. Intravenous diazepam is given to stop the fits, usually about 20–40 mg. This is followed in hospital by intravenous infusion of magnesium sulphate. This drug has been used for more than 60 years in the USA to prevent and treat eclamptic convulsions but has only recently found favour in the UK. It is thought to have central anticonvulsant activity. Clinical experience and research support its use in the prevention of subsequent eclamptic fits. It is usually given for at least 24 hours following the fit. Care must be taken as respiratory depression and loss of patellar reflexes may indicate toxicity.

Should the blood pressure be steeply raised, intravenous hydralazine is also given, either in a 5 mg bolus over 20 minute intervals or given intravenously as 25 mg in 500 ml of Hartmann's solution, with the drip rate titrated against the woman's blood pressure. This is best administered through a separate drip set so that magnesium sulphate and antihypertension treatments can be given at different rates

---

Box 9.2 Symptoms and signs of imminent eclampsia

- Upper abdominal pain
- Itching on the face
- Flashes of light
- Headache
- Rapidly increasing blood pressure
- Increasing proteinuria
- Increased knee jerks—hyper-reflexia

Box 9.3 Treatment of eclampsia

- Lie the woman on her side in the recovery position
- Keep airway clear
- Prevent trauma during fits
- Give diazepam immediately
- Give IV hydralazine if blood pressure is raised
- Give IV magnesium sulphate
- Use epidural anaesthesia if the woman is in labour or a caesarean section is planned

---

Box 9.4 Mode of delivery after control of eclampsia

- Factors favouring vaginal delivery
  - Multiparous mother
  - Stable blood pressure and diminished cerebral irritability
  - Ripe cervix
  - Mature fetus (>1500 g estimated weight)
  - Cephalic presentation
  - Normally grown fetus
  - Fetus in good state to stand uterine contractions

- Factors favouring caesarean section
  - Primiparous mother
  - Unstable blood pressure control or cerebral irritability
  - Unripe cervix
  - Immature fetus (<1500 g estimated weight)
  - Breech presentation
  - Intrauterine growth restriction
  - Poor prognosis of fetal state from Doppler blood flow rates or cardiotocography

according to clinical needs. If the woman is in labour or induction is considered, an epidural anaesthetic may be helpful, both to lower the blood pressure and to reduce the tendency to fit by removing the pain of intrauterine contractions. Any tendency of the woman to have disordered blood clotting should be excluded before insertion of a regional anaesthetic.

The ultimate treatment of eclampsia is delivery. Should eclampsia occur at home the woman must be transported to hospital immediately. Although rare, eclampsia still occurs in this country and the triennium 1994–96 was associated with 8 maternal deaths in the UK.

Timing of delivery

It must be emphasised that the ultimate cure of pregnancy-induced hypertension and eclampsia is delivery. The obstetrician must weigh the answers to two often conflicting questions:

● When would it be safer for the mother to be delivered?
● When would it be safer for the baby to be outside the uterus rather than on the wrong side of a failing placental exchange system?

Maternal considerations may be judged by the speed of deterioration of the condition (blood pressure and proteinuria) and the expected proximity of severe complications such as eclampsia. Fetal state is best evaluated by assessing the circulation supplying the fetus both in the spiral arteries with Doppler ultrasound measurements coming to the placental bed and in the umbilical vessels (discussed in Chapter 4). If there is time, serial ultrasound measurements of fetal growth are useful. If these data are available a rational decision can be made about the timing of the removal of the fetus from the hostile environment in a hospital with a neonatal intensive care unit. Women should be transferred early to regional centres for hypertension in pregnancy when it is obvious that the pregnancy-induced hypertension is not going to settle with bedrest and mild or moderate drug treatments. There is little place for heroic management in peripheral hospitals of a greatly compromised baby and mother.

Once it has been decided that it would be safer for the mother and the baby that delivery should occur the method and route of that delivery should be considered. If it is thought unsafe for the baby to undergo the contractions of labour, or if the baby is immature or has an inappropriate presentation, a caesarean section is indicated. If the mother's condition is deteriorating rapidly, again, the abdominal route would be swifter. An unripe cervix or an unsatisfactory presentation would also be grounds for a caesarean section. If, however, the woman has a ripe cervix, the hypertensive state is not worsening rapidly, and the fetus is in an acceptable position and of reasonable maturity, induction of labour should be performed with prostaglandin pessaries or membrane rupture, depending on the usage in the individual labour ward.

Intrauterine growth restriction is associated with pregnancy-induced hypertension. The two go together and share common causes. Narrowing of the placental bed vessels reduces nutrition to the fetus in pregnancy just as it reduces available oxygen during labour. Many fetuses born to women with unmanaged pregnancy-induced hypertension are small for their gestational age. Unfortunately so are many fetuses born to women who are very well managed; the fetal growth restriction therefore probably starts long before conventional management of the mother.

The ultimate treatment of eclampsia is delivery.

Maternal and fetal factors must be considered to find the best time for delivery of the fetus.

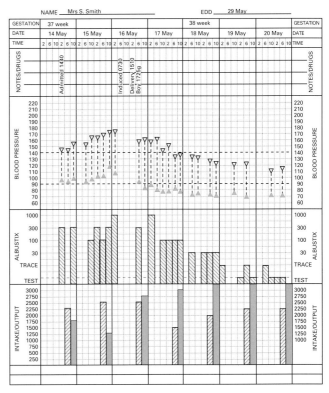

Figure 9.8 Partogram of a woman with severe pregnancy-induced hypertension before and after delivery

Box 9.5 Method of delivery (%) after various onsets of labour in women with pregnancies complicated by hypertension

● Spontaneous onset
 • Normal delivery – 3%
 • Vaginal operative delivery – 5%
 • Caesarean section – 10%

● Induced labour
 • Normal delivery – 17%
 • Vaginal operative delivery – 23%
 • Caesarean section – 22%

● Elective caesarean section – 11%

Conclusion

Pregnancy-induced hypertension is still a major problem in antenatal medicine but many of its worst effects can be mitigated by early diagnosis from blood pressure readings at clinic visits. The future includes predictive Doppler measurements of blood flow and preventive treatment, which may include aspirin, although the results of the CLASP trial in the United Kingdom are disappointing. If the condition is severe the mother's and baby's prognoses will be greatly improved if a regional hypertension in pregnancy unit is used.

Early diagnosis can modify some effects of pregnancy-induced hypertension.

References

1 CLASP. A randomised trial of low dose aspirin for the prevention and treatment of pre-eclampsia. *Lancet* 1994;**343**:619–29.
2 Eclampsia Trial Collaborative Group. Which anticonvulsant for women with eclampsia? *Lancet* 1995;**345**:1455–63.

Recommended reading

● Broughton Pipkin F. The hypertensive disorders of pregnancy. *Br Med J* 1995;**311**:609–13.
● Duley L. Anticonvulsants for the treatment of eclampsia. In: *Yearbook of obstetrics and gynaecology*, vol 5. London: RCOG Press, 1997.
● RCOG. *Management of eclampsia.* Guidelines no. 10. London: RCOG, 1999.

The figure showing transfer of glucose is reproduced by permission of Blackwell Scientific Publications from *Modern antenatal care of the fetus* edited by G Chamberlain and that showing change in plasma urate concentrations by permission of Churchill Livingstone from *Turnbull's obstetrics* edited by G Chamberlain.

10 Antepartum haemorrhage

Antepartum haemorrhage is bleeding from the genital tract between 24 completed weeks of pregnancy and the onset of labour. Some of the causes exist before this time and can produce bleeding. Although strictly speaking such bleeding is not an antepartum haemorrhage, the old fashioned definition is not appropriate for modern neonatal management.

The placental bed is the commonest site of antepartum haemorrhage; but in a few cases bleeding is from local causes in the genital tract. In a substantial remainder the bleeding may have no obvious cause but is probably still from the placental bed.

Placental abruption

If the placenta separates before delivery, the denuded placental bed bleeds. If the placenta is implanted in the upper segment of the uterus the bleeding is termed an abruption; if a part of the placenta is in the lower uterine segment it is designated a placenta praevia.

Placental abruption may entail only a small area of placental separation. The clot remains between placenta and placental bed but little or no blood escapes through the cervix (concealed abruption). Further separation causes further loss of blood, which oozes between the membranes and decidua, passing down through the cervix to appear at the vulva (revealed abruption).

In addition, the vessels around the side of the placenta may tear (marginal vein bleeding), which is clinically indistinguishable from placental abruption. The differentiation between revealed and concealed abruption is not very useful. The important factor is the amount of placenta separated from its bed and the coincident spasm in the surrounding placental bed vessels. If the area of separation and the proportion of placental bed vessels driven into spasm is sufficient, it will lead to fetal death.

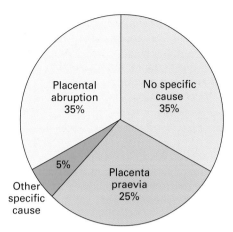

Figure 10.1 Causes of antepartum haemorrhage

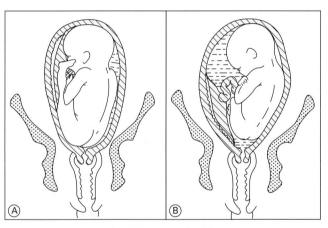

Figure 10.2 Placenta sited in (A) upper and (B) lower segment

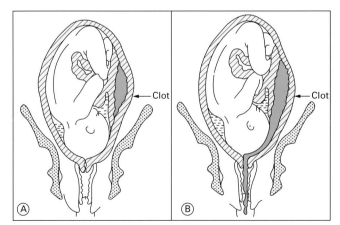

Figure 10.3 (A) Concealed and (B) revealed abruption from a normally sited placental bed

Pathology

Bleeding between the placenta and its bed causes separation; as more blood is forced between the layers, detachment becomes wider. Blood also tracks between the myometrial fibres, sometimes reaching the peritoneal surface. The mother's pain and shock depend on the amount of tissue damage rather than on the volume of bleeding. The fetal state depends on both the

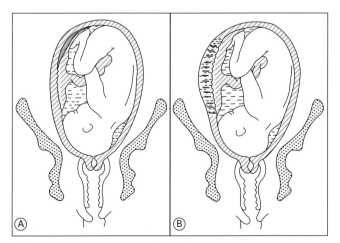

Figure 10.4 The degree of fetal effect depends on the amount of separation and spasm of placental bed vessels (A), while the maternal effect depends on the amount of tissue damage to the myometrium (B)

amount of separation and the spasm of the more peripheral blood vessels in the placental bed.

Sometimes amniotic fluid or trophoblast tissue is forced into the maternal circulation after a placental abruption. Thromboplastins start disseminated intravascular coagulation, which in a mild case is coped with by the maternal fibrinolytic system, but if an amniotic fluid embolus is large, maternal plasma fibrinogen concentration is depleted. Uterine bleeding continues with activation of the maternal fibrinolytic system; widespread deprivation of fibrin and fibrinogen follows, producing a vicious circle of more bleeding.

The cause of placental abruption is unknown. It happens more commonly in association with a uterine abnormality and there is a 10% risk of recurrence if it has occurred previously. Conditions of uterine overstretch such as twin pregnancy are associated with higher rates of abruption if amniotic fluid is released suddenly at the rupture of the membranes. Abdominal trauma is a less common association.

Diagnosis

The woman presents with poorly localised abdominal pain over the uterus; there may be some dark red vaginal bleeding or clots. Depending on the degree of placental separation, uterine spasm, and the loss of circulating blood into the tissue space, clinical shock may also be present. If the abruption is severe the uterus contracts tonically so that fetal parts cannot be felt; the fetus may be dead with no fetal heart detectable. Ultrasonography may show the retroplacental clot but gives no measure of the extent of functional disorder.

The differential diagnosis is from:

- Placenta praevia, which is not usually accompanied by pain, often results in brighter red bleeding as the blood is fresher and rarely results in so much shock.
- Rupture of the uterus, which may present with a similar picture to that of placental abruption.
- Red degeneration of a uterine fibroid at 24–30 weeks' gestation.
- Bleeding from a ruptured vessel on the surface of the pregnant uterus, which is rare.

The diagnosis of abruption is finally confirmed after delivery by finding organized clot firmly adherent to the placenta.

Management

A woman with an abruption is in a potentially dangerous condition and requires all the facilities the emergency services can provide. She must be admitted to hospital quickly. Group O rhesus negative blood may rarely be required urgently in the home but even if not, supportive intravenous treatment should be established. Hartmann's solution or saline may be used at first followed by a commercial plasma expander such as Haemaccel. Pain may be relieved by morphine, and the woman must be transferred to hospital, escorted by her GP, trained paramedic staff or the Flying Squad, when her condition is stable.

In hospital the antishock measures will be continued and blood given. At least six units of blood must be crossmatched, irrespective of the scant external blood loss; fresh frozen plasma and platelets should be available. Central venous pressures are a guide to the amount of blood required to prevent undertransfusion before delivery or overtransfusion afterwards. Once the condition is stabilised delivery should take place immediately. If the fetus is still alive, this could mean a caesarean section. This can be a difficult operation needing a

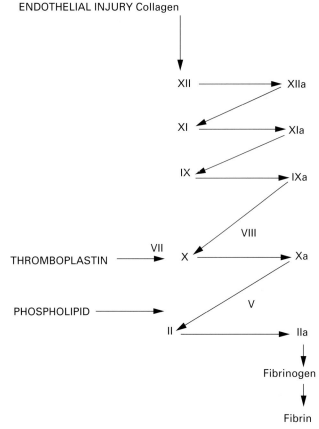

Figure 10.5 Points in the clotting cascade at which the sequelae of a placental abruption can intervene and so lead to disseminated intravascular coagulopathy

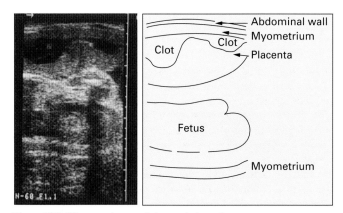

Figure 10.6 Ultrasound scan of placental abruption

Box 10.1   Management of placental abruption

- Get the woman to hospital urgently
- Replace volume of blood estimated lost from circulation rather than that seen at external loss
- Monitor central venous pressure
- Check for disseminated intravascular coagulopathy
- Check renal function and urinary output
- If fetus alive and mature, Caesarean section
- If fetus dead, induce (artificial rupture of the membranes)

senior obstetrician. If the fetus is dead, induction by rupture of the membranes usually leads to a rapid labour.

After a mild abruption and if the fetus is immature and lives the woman may continue the pregnancy under controlled conditions. She should stay in hospital with antenatal monitoring until the fetus is mature enough for delivery. In cases occurring very early in gestation the woman may have to be transferred for delivery to a regional unit with intensive neonatal facilities available.

Severe abruption may lead to severely disordered blood clotting which must be managed with the help of a haematologist. After delivery fluid balance should be carefully managed and urine output must be recorded hourly. Oliguria following reduced plasma volume is usually the result of acute tubular necrosis, though in rare cases acute cortical necrosis may occur. The help of anaesthetists trained in intensive care and of a renal physician will be needed.

Placenta praevia

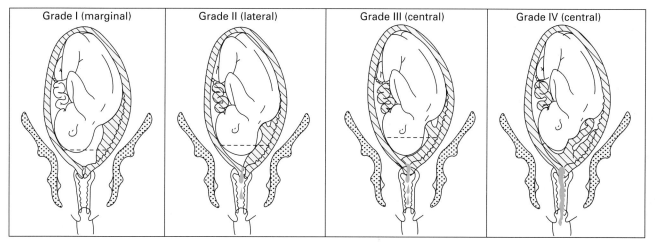

Figure 10.7 The older grades of placenta praevia were 1–4. They are now described in three grades: marginal, lateral, and central

The blastocyst usually implants in the thicker, receptive endometrium of the upper uterus, but occasionally it glissades to the endometrium of the isthmus or over a previous lower segment uterine scar. Then invasion by the trophoblast secures the embryo and when the uterus grows to form a lower segment later in pregnancy some part of the placenta is implanted there.

About a quarter of all antepartum haemorrhages are due to placenta praevia, the proportion increasing with more thorough investigative ultrasonography. In the last weeks of pregnancy the lower segment stretches whereas the placenta is comparatively inelastic. In consequence, the placenta which has implanted in the lower segment is peeled off the uterine wall with bleeding from the placental bed. A placenta praevia may be detected by ultrasonography in the mid-trimester but usually little bleeding occurs until the lower segment is formed after the 30th week.

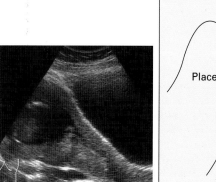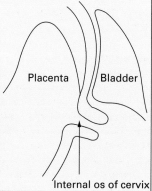

Figure 10.8 Ultrasound scan of placenta praevia

Diagnosis

A woman with placenta praevia may have bright red, painless vaginal bleeding. It comes unexpectedly, blood often being found on waking in the morning. The woman is in no way shocked and may wish to ignore the symptom as she feels normal.

A few women present with a persistent transverse lie or breech presentation in late pregnancy. The possibility of placenta praevia should always be considered in such a case and an ultrasound scan requested urgently. The result may lead little the woman's admission to hospital, even if she has had little bleeding.

In a third group of women a placenta praevia is diagnosed incidentally on ultrasound examination. This finding is common in the middle weeks of pregnancy. A low lying placenta diagnosed at 22 weeks' gestation is often normally sited by 32 weeks. About 5% of women present with a low lying placenta at 24 weeks but only 1% of them have a placenta praevia at term. The upper segment of the uterus grows and the placental site moves with it as the lower segment is formed. If not, such women should be treated in the same way as others diagnosed clinically because the risk of bleeding in late pregnancy is as great.

The uterine spasm of placental abruption does not occur in placenta praevia and the fetus can be felt easily. The fetus is usually alive with a good heart beat. The woman's degree of shock will vary directly with the amount of blood lost. If shock is moderate the woman needs admission to hospital. If blood loss is slight she can go to the hospital conventionally but she needs to be warned of the probable diagnosis.

No vaginal examinations should be performed on any woman who bleeds in late pregnancy until a placenta praevia has been excluded by ultrasonography. If this principle is broached, further separation of the placenta may occur with very heavy, and sometimes fatal, haemorrhage. Any woman who presents to a general practitioner with vaginal bleeding in late pregnancy should be considered to have a placenta praevia until the diagnosis is disproved. She must be referred to a hospital for an urgent appointment that day. If necessary, she should be admitted if ultrasound investigations cannot be performed straight away.

In hospital blood is crossmatched and the placental site demonstrated by ultrasonography. The older diagnostic radioisotope studies and soft tissue x ray examinations now have no place in the UK.

Once placenta praevia is diagnosed, the aim of treatment is to maintain the pregnancy until the fetus is mature enough to be delivered; at 38 weeks an elective caesarean section will probably be performed unless the placenta praevia is a minor one with the fetal presenting part below it. Should the placenta be anterior, the descending fetal head may compress it against the back of the symphysis pubis, so allowing a vaginal delivery, but this is uncommon. The Caesarian operation may be difficult with much blood loss and should be performed by a senior obstetrician.

Other specific causes of bleeding

General
Few haemorrhagic diseases occur in young women but vaginal bleeding may occur in von Willebrand's disease, Hodgkin's disease, and leukaemia. All are probably known about beforehand, and the diagnosis is confirmed from the results of haematological studies.

Local
Lesions of the cervix and vagina cause slight bleeding, often only a smear of blood and mucus. Moderate bleeding may occur with a carcinoma of the cervix—unusual in women of childbearing age—or varicose veins of the vulva and lower vagina. Lesser bleeding is more likely from a polyp or an erosion of the cervix. Monilia infection may be accompanied by spotting as plaques of fungoid tissue are separated from the vaginal walls.

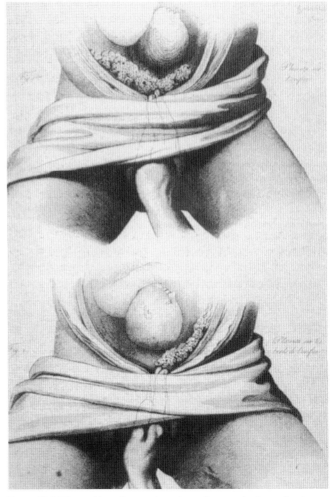

Figure 10.9 These old steel engravings show what a vaginal examination could do to a placenta praevia (central (above) and lateral (below)). NEVER DO A VAGINAL EXAMINATION UNLESS PLACENTA PRAEVIA HAS BEEN EXCLUDED

Table 10.1 Causes of antepartum bleeding from the lower genital tract

Cause	Characteristic bleeding
Cervical ectropion	Smear of blood loss often with mucous loss
Cervical polyp	Spotting of blood
Cervical cancer	Smear of blood on touch (rare, but diagnosis is important)
	May bleed heavily
Vaginal infection	Spotting of blood with white or pink discharge
Vaginal varicose veins	Occasionally heavy bleeding

All these causes can be diagnosed by using a speculum, but this procedure must be done in hospital after the woman has been assessed and ultrasound examination has excluded placenta praevia. If the haemorrhage is due to a benign local lesion it will be managed appropriately.

Fetal

A most unusual cause of bleeding is from fetal blood vessels. There may be a succenturiate lobe or the umbilical cord may be inserted into the membranes over the internals so that the arteries and veins pass unsupported to reach the edge of the placenta. If by chance the placenta is also low lying, the umbilical blood vessels pass over the internal os of the cervix (vasa praevia); when the membranes rupture the fetal vessels may tear and bleed. The blood is fetal and a small loss can lead to severe hypovolaemia of the fetus.

The presence of vasa praevia is difficult to diagnose but sometimes they can be suspected with colour Doppler ultrasonography. More usually the fetal heart rate may alter abruptly after membrane rupture accompanied by a very slight blood loss. Bedside tests exist to differentiate fetal from maternal haemoglobin but are rarely used. The treatment must be a rapid caesarean section as the fetus cannot stand such blood loss for long.

Bleeding of unknown origin

The real cause of antepartum haemorrhage is unknown in a large number of women. They may have bled from separation of the lower part of a normally sited placental bed or the membranes may have sheared with tearing of very small blood vessels. Some placentas bleed early from their edge.

If the cause of antepartum haemorrhage cannot be diagnosed precisely, the woman should not be dismissed lightly. The risk to her baby at subsequent labour is higher than background, although the risk to the mother does not seem to be great. It is good practice to keep such women in hospital for some days, allowing them to return home if no further vaginal bleeding occurs. This rule of thumb seems to cover most eventualities and so many women do not stay in hospital for long. Fetal growth should be monitored by ultrasonography. In labour, however, the fetus should be monitored for hypoxia: for there is a higher risk than in fetuses whose mothers have not bled.

Recommended reading

- Barron F, Hill W. Placenta praevia, placental abruption. *Clin Obstet Gynaecol* 1998;**41**:527–32.
- Bonner J. Massive obstetric haemorrhage. *Best Pract Clin Obstet Gynaecol* 2000;**14**:1–16.
- RCOG. *Placenta praevia: diagnosis and management. Guidelines no. 27.* London: RCOG, 2001.

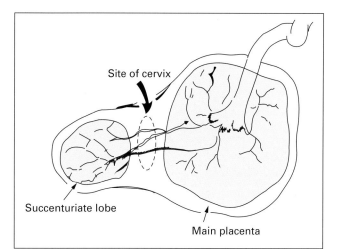

Figure 10.10 Vasa praevia. A succenturiate lobe is separated from the main body of the placenta. Should the vessels run over the cervix, when the cervix dilates they may be torn so that fetal blood is lost

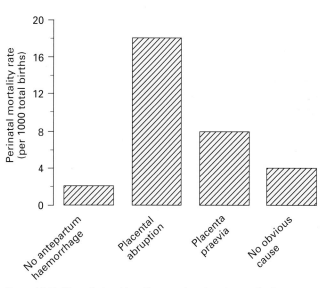

Figure 10.11 The relative risks of increased perinatal mortality from antepartum haemorrhage compared with those in pregnancies with no such haemorrhage

11 Small for gestational age

The problems of small babies and preterm labour often go together and are now the major causes of perinatal mortality and morbidity in the UK. Furthermore, they use up large amounts of facilities, manpower, and finance. Preterm labour and premature rupture of the membranes are considered in the next chapter and the antenatal care of fetuses that are small for gestational age and of their mothers in this one.

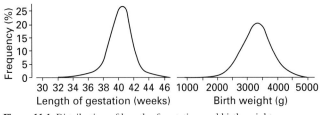

Figure 11.1 Distribution of length of gestation and birth weight (singletons, last menstrual period certain)

The diagnosis of a small fetus is made more specific by examining the ratio of birth weight (or estimated birth weight) to gestational age. Both these measures have inherent problems.

Obstetricians estimate fetal weight either clinically or from measuring ultrasound determined diameters of the fetus *in utero*. Gestational age is derived from the mother's menstrual dates, which are usually confirmed by an ultrasound scan measuring the biparietal diameter performed before 20 weeks. In most parts of the UK, about 80% of women are sure of their dates. The figure shows the distribution of length of gestation for women according to whether they were sure of their dates. The frequency of heavier babies was increased among those uncertain of the date of their last menstrual period. All women in the UK with unsure dates should have gestational age established by ultrasound, as should those in whom there is a discrepancy between the dates derived from the last menstrual period and fetal size in early pregnancy. Obstetricians consider a baby to be small for gestational age when abdominal circumference readings fall below the second standard deviation below the mean; this is approximately the second centile on serial ultrasonography.

After birth paediatricians can weigh the baby and so have a precise measure, although even this varies slightly with the conditions of weighing and when it is done. Gestational age is obtained from the obstetrician by one of the previously mentioned measures or from Dubowitz scoring. The data are plotted on a specific centile chart; various groups of paediatricians take small for gestational age as being below the 10th, the fifth, or the third centile. It is very important when examining data to know which of these measures was used. The 10th centile is rather crude and will include many normal babies at the lower end of the normal birthweight distribution curves whose growth has not actually been affected by placental bed disease.

Much simpler was the old measure of prematurity, taking a cut off point of a birth weight of less than 2500 g. Unfortunately, this includes small babies whose birth weight is appropriate for their gestational age and those who are small for their gestational age, two very different groups in clinical medicine. For example, babies born with a birth weight below

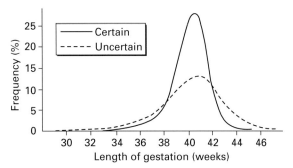

The phrase "intrauterine retardation" is no longer used in current obstetrics. It has been replaced by "intrauterine growth restriction" because the former phrase implied that there was some retardation of the child, particularly cerebral, and some parents found this difficult to accept.

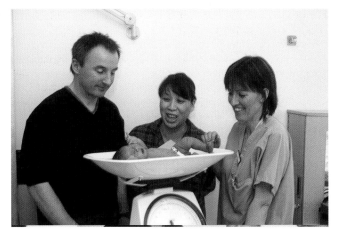

Figure 11.2 Distribution of length of gestation by knowledge of last menstrual period (singletons)

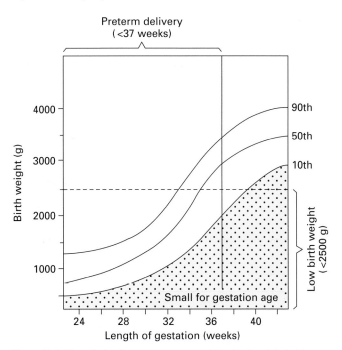

Figure 11.3 Weighing a newborn

Figure 11.4 The relation between preterm and low birth weight babies. Babies who are small for gestational age fall under the 10th centile

2500 g make up about 7% of the newborn population in the UK, about 3% in Sweden, almost 11% in Hungary and a much higher proportion in many parts of the Eastern hemisphere. Such mixed data would make a nonsense of studying the influences on fetal growth and so the definition of small for gestational age relating birth weight to length of intrauterine life stands at the moment.

Causes

Genetic abnormalities

Genetic abnormalities are an identifiable but not very common factor causing growth restriction. Trisomy 21 is the commonest example, though osteogenesis imperfecta, Potter's syndrome, and anencephaly may all be associated with intrauterine growth restriction. Other congenital malformations not yet proved to have a genetic component are commonly found in fetuses that are small for gestational age; among them are gastrointestinal abnormalities such as atresia of the duodenum, gastroschisis, and omphalocele.

Maternal nutrition

In the UK the effect of maternal nutrition on low birth weight is probably small. Extremes of starvation associated with small babies are rare in Britain. During a pregnancy about 80 000 kilocalories (335 MJ) of extra energy is required, of which 36 000 kilocalories (150 MJ) is for maintenance metabolism.[1] Much of this can come from an everyday diet, and among well nourished women requirements change little for the first 10 weeks of pregnancy. Thence requirements gradually increase, but ordinary variations in food intake are unlikely to affect events. It is unwise to recommend that a mother eat for two in order to produce a larger baby. As well as the nutritional value of the food consumed, there are other factors of appetite, maternal obesity, and heartburn which must be remembered when making recommendations.

Intrauterine infection

Most intrauterine infections are viral or bacterial. Some 60% of babies with congenital rubella are born below the 10th centile of weight for gestation. Cytomegalovirus and toxoplasmosis (much less common in this country than in mainland Europe) are associated with growth restriction in about 40% of infected infants. Malaria, ubiquitous in many tropical countries, causes a massive accumulation of monocytes in the intravillus space, which is associated with a fetus being small for gestational age.

Drugs

Drugs may be a cause of babies being small for gestational age. The commonest cases in the UK are the results of tobacco fumes being absorbed during cigarette smoking. The association between smoking and small for gestational age babies is well documented. The number of affected babies whose growth drops below the 10th centile increases during the last weeks of gestation.

The effect of alcohol is difficult to sort out. At the extreme end of the range, i.e. women drinking more than 45 units of alcohol a week, some babies are born with the fetal alcohol syndrome and a distinctly reduced birth weight. At lower intakes of alcohol covariables come into play; a deficient maternal diet and increased cigarette smoking are often associated with the alcohol habit. In some studies multivariant analyses show that the main causal factor associated with low birth weight is not alcohol intake but cigarette smoking. The whole lifestyle is probably the important factor. Some doctors

In the UK most of the energy required by a pregnant woman can come from an ordinary diet, with little need for supplementation.

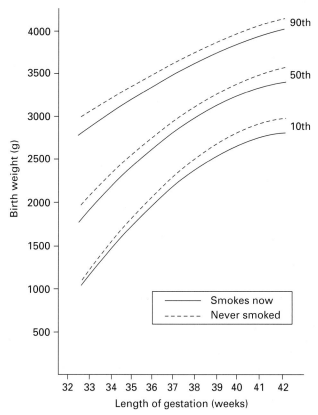

Figure 11.5 Centiles of birth weight by length of gestation and mother's smoking habit (singletons, last menstrual period certain)

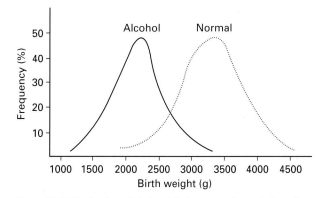

Figure 11.6 Distribution of birth weight in a normal population of women and in one consisting of women who drank more than 45 units of alcohol a week (heavy drinking)

consider that smoking in pregnancy is the most important single cause of low birth weight, the greatest single factor associated with death and illness in the first weeks of life.

The use of narcotic drugs is commonly associated with low birth weight but, again, the total lifestyle of the woman may be the real factor. For this reason, perhaps, an increased incidence of small for gestational age babies persists with methadone users.

Therapeutic drugs such as carbamazepine and the valproates have been associated with an increased incidence of small for gestational age babies, as have the more powerful antiviral drugs such as azathioprine. Such powerful drugs are not given in pregnancy unless they are needed to treat a serious maternal medical condition, which in itself may affect nutrition or metabolism of the mother and therefore growth of the fetus.

Hypertension

One of the major current causes of babies being small for gestational age in the UK is hypertension in the mother, either pregnancy induced or pre-existing. After other features have been taken into account such types of hypertension are associated with about a third of all cases of intrauterine growth restriction. The effects of hypertension are made worse when raised blood pressure is associated with proteinuria, implying a greater reduction of the maternal perfusion of the placental bed. The duration of the condition also has an effect; for example, 80% of mothers who have proteinuric pregnancy-induced hypertension before the 34th week of pregnancy have infants with a birth weight below the 10th centile.

Other factors

The maternal body habitus is not a major factor in babies being small for gestational age, but big women do produce larger children. The father's influence is less important, classically shown in the 1938 study of Walton and Hammond on Shire horses and Shetland ponies.[2]

The altitude at which a woman lives in pregnancy has a negative effect on fetal growth, particularly if she is not used to high altitudes.

Diagnosis

Extreme examples of fetuses that are severely small for gestational age can sometimes be diagnosed by palpation. This is most likely if the same midwife or doctor sees the woman at each antenatal visit and uses the written records of previous visits longitudinally. In several control studies false positive rates as high as 50% and low predictive values have been found in the clinical estimation of intrauterine growth restriction.

The use of symphysio-fundal height measurements is probably of more use in detecting the large baby or polyhydramnios than the small baby or oligohydramnios. A randomised trial of symphysio-fundal height mesurements was able to detect fewer small for gestational age fetuses by this method, 28% compared with 48% in the palpation group without measuring fundal height.[3]

Sometimes the lack of amniotic fluid is diagnosed more readily; oligohydramnios accompanies fetuses that are small for gestational age and therefore may lead to ultrasound investigation more swiftly than when fetal size has been estimated clinically.

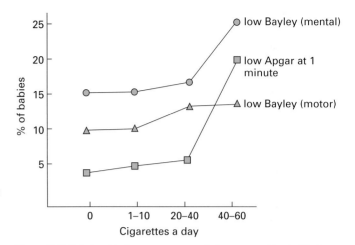

Figure 11.7 Relationship between amount of cigarette smoking in black American women and various non-weight related indices at birth and seven months later

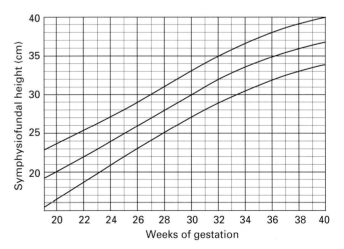

Figure 11.8 The effects of sire and mare on the size of offspring are shown in this 1938 experiment in which Shire horses and Shetland ponies were mated. The maternal influence predominates

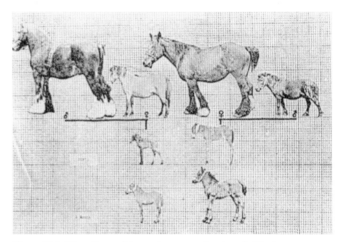

Figure 11.9 Mean (± SD) of symphysio-fundal height by weeks of gestation. Note the wide range of readings for any given week of gestation and the even wider range of expected gestation weeks for any given reading

Most fetuses that are small for gestational age are diagnosed in this country by ultrasound. When a good estimate of gestational age in early pregnancy has been obtained and fetal abnormalities have been excluded, ultrasound scans can give valuable measures of fetal growth. Scans of the abdominal circumference at the level of the umbilical vessels give a measure of liver growth. Another measure of somatic growth is femur length.

Fetuses with small abdominal circumferences can have their head circumference measured and the ratio of head to abdominal circumference derived. A small for gestational age fetus with a normal ratio of head to abdominal circumference tends to be a perfect miniature (bonsai baby) and is usually normal, representing the lower end of biological variation. Such fetuses, however, may also be associated with chromosomal anomalies, drugs, infection, and malnutrition.

Fetuses suffering from placental bed malperfusion tend to preserve growth of the head at the expense of the body because a protective mechanism shunts blood to the brain. Measuring the ratio of head circumference to abdominal circumferences can sometimes differentiate those that are just normally small (normal ratio) and those that are growth restricted (increased ratio).

Occasionally there may be a chromosomal reason for the poor growth picture and an ultrasound assessment may help determine if a karyotype is indicated. Structural anomalies such as cardiac defects, dilated renal pelves, or abnormal head shapes may be suggestive. Alternatively a history of maternal infection or increased viral antibodies may point to an infective cause.

All small babies require close assessment. Estimating fetal weight should include serial ultrasound including measurements, liquor volume, and Doppler studies of the umbilical artery. Cardiotography is used to give reassurance especially if there is doubt about fetal movements.

Small for gestational age fetuses may be screened by using early ultrasound to confirm gestational age and later to confirm growth. Finer tuning is possible by Doppler measurement of the afferent blood supply to the placental bed, with later changes in blood velocity along the umbilical vessels giving a more precise warning of fetal state. Should the umbilical artery end diastolic frequencies be lost, delivery should be considered very soon, provided pregnancy is far enough advanced that the neonatal unit of the hospital concerned is happy to deal with a child of that gestation.

In the past, most babies had ultrasound reading of the biparietal diameter at 16–20 weeks to confirm gestation and a second scan of abdominal circumference at 32–36 weeks to check growth. The later scan is now more commonly done only on suspicion of poor fetal growth and has been dispensed with in most UK obstetric departments.

Mothers whose fetuses are at greater risk of intrauterine growth restriction often have several ultrasound readings performed in later pregnancy. Such women include those with a history of perinatal death and of intrauterine growth restriction previously as well as those in whom the fetus is exposed to some of the aetiological factors already considered and where oligohydramnios may give a clue.

Treatment

The ultimate treatment of a fetus with impaired growth associated with an abnormal placental bed is delivery. Diagnosis encapsulates the fact that a baby getting insufficient nutrition

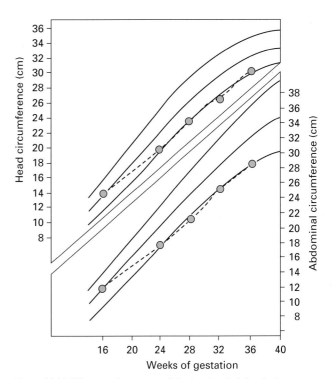

Figure 11.10 Ultrasound measures of the head and abdominal circumference. Although growth rates are diminished, they fall at the same rate—symmetrical growth restriction

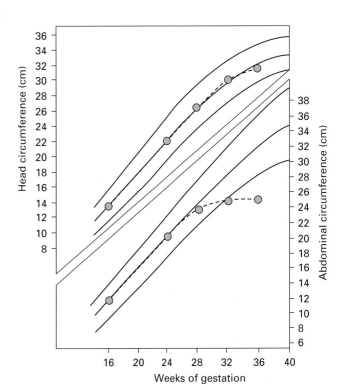

Figure 11.11 Ultrasound measures of head and abdominal circumference. Abdominal growth slows more than head growth—asymmetrical growth restriction

for normal growth will be in greater danger of oxygen deprivation in labour. Removal from the hostile environment would be the ultimate answer, but this might not be wise in earlier gestation (24–28 weeks); efforts are made to improve the blood supply to the placental bed.

Rest, particularly with the woman lying on her left side for some hours a day, should theoretically improve placental perfusion, but Doppler studies show little evidence for its effectiveness. Measures to restore the plasma volume and to give adequate hydration may be useful theoretically as they should decrease viscosity and lead to an improvement of intrauterine blood flow. Again, theory is not matched by practice.

In fetuses that are small for gestational age, correction and reversal of some of the causal factors might have helped, but it is too late to do this when the fetus is detectably small for gestational age. For example, curtailment of cigarette smoking should happen in early pregnancy. Such reduction in the first 16 weeks allows fetuses to follow a normal growth pattern rather than that of growth restricted babies of smoking mothers.

The mother of a fetus that is small for gestational age should attend a hospital with the capacity for more precise diagnosis and where special ultrasound and Doppler measurements are available. Many tertiary referral centres have a fetal assessment unit run on a day care basis. Women who live near large hospitals with such facilities can still be outpatients while having full surveillance. If they live away from the centre, however, they may have to be transferred and become inpatients; this is the keystone of the *in utero* transfer system widespread in the UK. Probably a third of the women admitted as *in utero* transfers have fetuses that are small for gestational age as their indication for admission.

The ultrasound surveillance of fetal growth, liquor volume, and umbilical vessel blood flow allows more precise fetal prognosis. Prospective frequent and regular consultations with the neonatal paediatrician who will be involved are essential. This will help to prepare for a premature delivery. The mother is also given steroids to reduce the risk of respiratory distress syndrome in her baby.

The fetus must be delivered at the most appropriate time by the most appropriate method. The time depends on weighing up the risks of keeping the fetus inside the uterus, that is, those of diminished placental bed perfusion, against the risks of being outside, that is, the risks of immaturity and survival in a good intensive care neonatal unit. The critical gestational age for these decisions is being pushed back all the time; now the worrying time for most obstetricians and neonatal paediatricians is 24–28 weeks. Once a pregnancy passes 28 weeks the concern is much less, although the respiratory distress syndrome can still cause morbidity and even death after delivery, especially in those small for gestational age.

The next time

Studies of pregnancies subsequent to one producing a small for gestational age baby showed that growth restriction only recurs in 20% and when it did it was less severe. In consequence, although this gives a better prognosis, it makes any management plans hard to assess for four-fifths of women will not get the problem anyway in the next pregnancy, prevention measures used prospectively thus may not have been needed. Even harder is research; use of paired studies with controls or randomised controlled trials is essential.

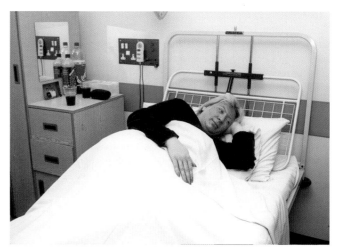

Figure 11.12 Woman lying in the left lateral position

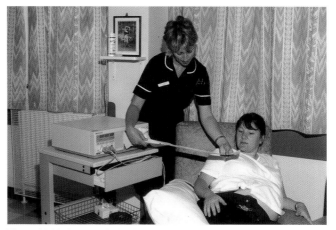

Figure 11.13 Corner of a fetal assessment unit

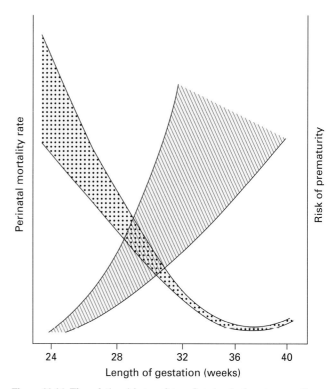

Figure 11.14 The relative risks to a fetus of staying in the uterus on the wrong side of a poor placental bed perfusion system ⋯ compared with the risks of being delivered too soon ▨

Conclusion

It must be remembered that the definitions of small for gestational age are used imprecisely and much that was thought to be known about its causation depended on data that were not mutually comparable. Until Doppler measurement, the measures of fetal wellbeing were also inexact; even Doppler ultrasound is not the last word on the subject. The ultimate management depends on avoiding trouble. Maybe we are overprotective of fetuses that are small for gestational age, but it is the best that we can do in 2001.

> The diagnosis, causes, and management of small for gestational age fetuses are all still uncertain. The best management is prevention.

Recommended reading

- Nathanidez P, Smith G. Regulation of the myometrium in term and preterm labour. In O'Brien P, ed. *Yearbook of obstetrics and gynaecology*, no. 8. London: RCOG, 2000.
- Robinson J, Hok F, Decker G. Intrauterine growth restriction. In O'Brien P, ed. *Yearbook of obstetrics and gynaecology*, no. 8. London: RCOG, 2000.

References

1 Hytten FE. Nutrition. In: Hytten FE, Chamberlain G, eds. *Clinical physiology in obstetrics*. 2nd edn. Oxford: Blackwell Scientific Publications, 1990:150–72.
2 Walton A, Hammond J. The maternal effects on growth in Shire horses and Shetland pony crosses. *Proc Roy Soc London [Biol]* 1938;**125**:311–35.
3 Lindhard A, Nielson P, Mooritsen L, Zachariassen A, Sørensen H, Rosenø A. Implications of introducing symphysio-fundal height measurements. *Br J Obstet Gynaec* 1990;**97**:675.

The figures showing the distribution of birth weight, the distribution of the length of gestation, the centiles of birth weight by length of gestation and date of the last menstrual period, and the centiles of birth weight by length of gestation and maternal smoking habit are reproduced by permission of Butterworth Heinemann from *British Births 1970* by R Chamberlain and G Chamberlain; this is an account of the National Birthday Trust's 1970 study.

12 Preterm labour

Preterm labour may result in the birth of an immature infant. Together with intrauterine growth restriction it is the main problem of obstetric care in the UK. The conventional definition of preterm labour includes women delivering before 37 completed weeks of gestation, but in practice in the UK problems arise mostly with births before 34 weeks. Babies more mature than this can be cared for successfully in many district general hospitals without intensive care facilities; most problems arise in babies weighing less than 1500 g (3·5 lb).

Perinatal mortality rates relate sharply to maturity and birth weight; similarly, neonatal mortality rates relate to weight at birth. Probably some 6% of babies in the United Kingdom are born before 37 weeks and 2% before the 32nd week of pregnancy.

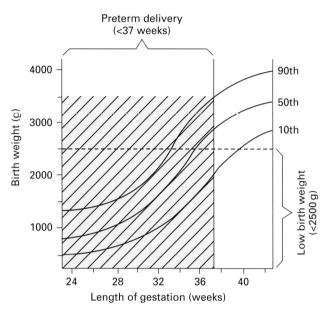

Figure 12.1 Relation between length of gestation and birth weight. Babies born in the crosshatched area are preterm irrespective of weight

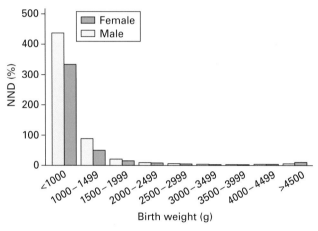

Figure 12.2 Neonatal deaths per 1000 live births by sex and birth weight, England and Wales 1995

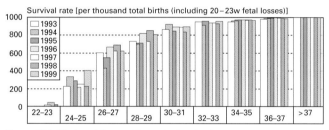

Figure 12.3 Birth weight specific survival to 28 days 1993–9 (Welsh Perinatal Survey)

Causes

Sociobiological background

The capacity for preterm labour is often predictable by a clustering of high risk factors. The mother's age, parity, and socioeconomic class bear strong associations with preterm labour. Socioeconomic class is an indicator of the woman's behaviour, nutrition, smoking, and previous preterm delivery. Also important is a woman's work in early pregnancy, particularly if it involves continuous standing. These may not be individual factors in their own right but are useful to identify women whose risk of preterm labour is increased.

Reproductive history

A multiparous woman's obstetric history may give prognostic clues; the chances of a preterm delivery are tripled after one previous preterm birth and increased sixfold after two. These are two simple sets of risks; other outcomes bring in differential variables. Past studies have been diminished by not including the woman's total obstetric history, which needs careful consideration in the case of each woman.

Medical history

Recurrent lower urinary tract infections are not usually associated with recurrent preterm labour, although pyelonephritis may be. The renal tract should be investigated

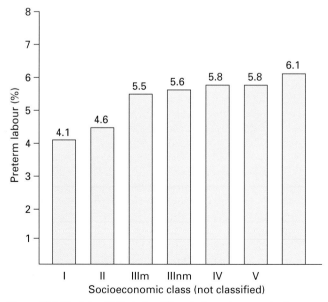

Figure 12.4 Singleton births before 37 weeks by socioeconomic class (Scotland 1990–95)

72

between pregnancies and reinfection prevented by prophylactic antibiotics in future pregnancies.

Uterine structural abnormalities can be a recurrent factor, the best documented being cervical incompetence. This follows damage or overstretch of the cervical internal os—an ill-formed muscular sphincter—and is a mechanical diagnosis first observed by obstetricians in the 1940s and made familiar by the work of Shirodkar and McDonald in the 1950s. The truer picture of the place of cervical incompetence and its management in preterm labour had to await a randomised controlled trial in the 1980s run jointly by the Medical Research Council and the Royal College of Obstetricians and Gynaecologists; the results put into proportion the importance of cervical incompetence as an individual factor in preterm delivery.[1] A much smaller report had more optimistic results (Table. 12.1).

Complications of pregnancy

Multiple pregnancy is a marker for preterm labour. The mean gestation of twins is 37 weeks and therefore many will be born before this time.

Several studies have shown the association of preterm labour with antepartum haemorrhage, irrespective of the cause of the bleeding.

Hard physical work in pregnancy is associated with preterm labour, particularly if it is repetitive and boring or in an unpleasant, noisy environment. This factor is discussed in Chapter 6.

Abnormalities of the fetus are often associated with preterm labour when there may also be polyhydramnios, which in itself can lead to premature membrane rupture and preterm labour.

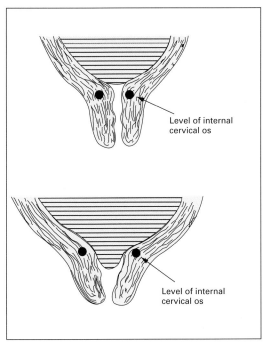

Figure 12.5 Cervical incompetence leads to a cone of unsupported membranes

Table 12.1 **Effectiveness of cervical cerclage in reducing preterm delivery and rates of stillbirth, miscarriage, and neonatal death[2]**

	No in group		Odds ratio and 95% confidence interval						
	Experimental	Control	0.01	0.1	0.5	1	2	10	100
Delivered:									
Before 33 weeks	59/454	82/451			●				
Before 37 weeks	124/454	146/451			●				
Stillbirth, miscarriage, or									
neonatal death	37/454	54/451			●				

Data analysed 1993.

Infection and premature membrane rupture

Infection of the lower uterus and the membranes is an important feature that is poorly investigated epidemiologically. The presence of micro-organisms in the membranes is associated with an increased production of prostaglandins, one of the main factors associated with the onset of labour. Proteases, coagulases, and elastases are also produced by invading micro-organisms, whose endotoxins may stimulate labour directly as well as through prostaglandin metabolism. Low grade chorioamnionitis (infection of the membranes) is much commoner after premature rupture of the membranes, when an ascending infection from the vagina may produce such biochemical changes. One of the commonest organisms is the β haemolytic streptococcus, which is found as a commensal in the vagina in about 5% of women but may be a factor in preterm labour in up to 20%. Other anaerobic vaginoses are more common in women with premature rupture of

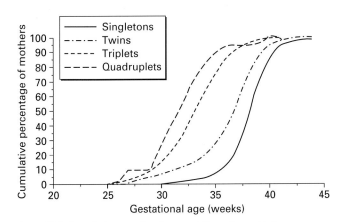

Figure 12.6 Cumulative gestational age at delivery for multiple pregnancies. By 37 weeks delivery has occurred in 97% of quadruplet, 96% of triplet, 55% of twin, and 25% of singleton pregnancies

ABC of Antenatal Care

membranes and preterm labour than in those who go to term. Changes in vaginal flora have been shown by culturing vaginal flora in mid-trimester and before labour. The persistence of *Bacteroides* in the last months of pregnancy was associated with preterm birth. Coliforms when associated with preterm labour were acquired later in pregnancy.[3] Premature membrane rupture itself is a commonly quoted cause of preterm labour; this may be due to the infection that weakened the forewaters or to the removal of the forewaters' mechanical support from the cervix.

Induction
Preterm labour is caused iatrogenically in about 15% of women in this country, though in some units the rate rises to 40%. Many of the inductions will obviously be in women after 37 weeks' gestation but some will be performed before this. The problem of rhesus incompatibility, previously a major indication, has reduced markedly; in its place is pregnancy-induced proteinuric hypertension and intrauterine growth restriction. Women with either of these problems should be delivered at hospitals that can cope with the neonatal sequelae of such induction; these groups produce a large proportion of babies who are born well before the 37th week of pregnancy.

Prevention
The recognition of some of the triggers of preterm labour has led some obstetricians to take action to prevent labour. There is little objective evidence that bedrest and the use of prophylactic tocolytic agents are helpful, although a doctor might use either of these managements to satisfy a mother who has previously undergone preterm labour and has faith in them. Repeated, carefully taken, high vaginal swabs to give the pattern of micro-organisms in the upper vagina may be useful. Active antibiotic treatment will eradicate colonisation and thus reduce the risks of preterm labour. Clindamycin is being used in this field and the whole approach is under evaluation.

Several centres have used programmes during early and mid-pregnancy to educate women with a history of preterm delivery to try to prevent a recurrence of the problem. There is no easy method of doing this in a group; the success of such programmes depends on the individual woman and her individual midwives and doctors. All the factors discussed so far must be considered, and the woman should obviously try to avoid those which seem to be the more relevant in her case. Even with the most intensive antenatal education programmes, preterm deliveries are not cut to less than about 3·5%, a background rate in many populations. Success in this subject may come eventually after a conscious effort to modify the lifestyle, socioeconomic conditions, and medical problems of each individual patient.

Diagnosis
As with labour at term, diagnosing the onset of preterm labour is more easily performed retrospectively than at the time. You can look back and say a labour probably started at a certain time, but to do so prospectively is much harder. The general practitioner is left with the difficult task of deciding whether any group of uterine contractions will progress to cervical dilatation or whether they are just stronger Braxton Hicks contractions. The diagnosis may be assisted by external tocographic measurement of uterine contractions with a semiquantitative external monitor. Any woman thought to be in preterm labour should go to the local maternity unit as soon as possible for further assessment. There tocography may help, and assessment of the cervix may be valuable. About half of the women who present with regular, painful contractions will not

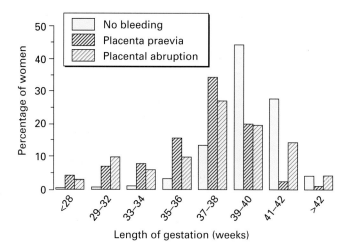

Figure 12.7 Time of delivery among women who had no vaginal bleeding in pregnancy compared with that among those with placenta praevia or placental abruption (n = 17 005)

Box 12.1 Major indications for induction of preterm labour
• Pregnancy-induced proteinuric hypertension
• Intrauterine growth restriction

Box 12.2 Prevention of preterm labour
• Control vaginal infection
• Education about early signs of labour
• Cervical cerclage (if relevant)
• ? Bedrest
• ? Prophylactic tocolytics
• Better control of conditions that would require early iatrogenic induction of labour

---

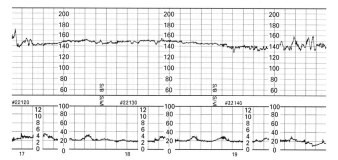

Figure 12.8 Cardiogram with fetal heart rate (above) and uterine pressure (below). The fetus is asleep for much of this trace and regular small contractions of the uterus are seen

74

progress to labour. Impending preterm labour may disrupt the cells of the cervix releasing fibronection. The cells can be detected fairly simply and are the basis of a test to check whether that woman is at risk of going into preterm labour soon. It is more useful in the early treatment of high-risk women but of less use in those at lower risk.

If preterm labour seems inevitable, treatment may be given to postpone it. Otherwise, the woman may be kept in for 24 hours to see if labour follows; if not, she can be discharged home to the care of her general practitioner. It is easy to be wise after the event, but only by sending every woman about whom there is reasonable doubt to the maternity unit will clinicians not miss the occasional woman who goes into very early preterm labour. Ultrasound evaluation of the cervix can sometimes warn of preterm labour. In some women dilatation, funnelling of the internal os and shortening of the canal all can be demonstrated but the specificity of the investigation is not high. A vaginal examination still gives the clearest evaluation of preterm labour.

Inhibition of established preterm labour
If a woman is in real preterm labour a decision has to be made whether labour should be stopped. It is probably wise not to do so if the mother's blood pressure is raised, there is proved infection in the endocervical or decidual regions, or the fetus has a lethal abnormality. Some obstetricians would consider further that it was unwise to inhibit labour in the presence of long-term rupture of the membranes, severe intrauterine growth restriction, or an antepartum haemorrhage. Each of these cases must be decided on their own merits.

Other than these exceptions, in most cases before 28 weeks it is worth trying to stop preterm labour to buy intrauterine time for the fetus. In the short term this can allow emergency treatment such as steroids to help maturation of the fetal respiratory system or allow transfer of the woman to a centre with good neonatal care facilities for a very small baby after delivery. These decisions must be made in consultation with the paediatricians as the practical management of any baby resulting from a preterm labour will depend on their skills and facilities. In a large well equipped obstetric-paediatric unit the borderline comes at about 27 weeks, provided that all other features of the pregnancy are normal.

If it is considered necessary to stop preterm labour a range of agents exist. Alcohol and the progestogens are obsolete.

Before 32 weeks' gestation short-term inhibition of labour allows:

- Transfer to the delivery unit best equipped for special neonatal care
- Steroids to be given to help mature the fetal respiratory system

A third of children born between 32 and 35 weeks' gestation may expect to have problems at school by the age of seven.

Table 12.2 Effectiveness of β mimetic tocolytics used in preterm labour in reducing preterm delivery. The numbers are the proportions of women delivering before 37 weeks[2]

Study	No in group		Odds ratio and 95% confidence interval
	Experimental	Control	
Christensen et al. (1980)	1/14	0/16	
Spellacy et al. (1979)	1/15	4/15	
Barden (unpublished)	1/12	0/13	
Hoebel (unpublished)	2/17	0/16	
Cotton et al. (1984)	1/19	4/19	
Howard et al. (1982)	1/16	1/21	
Ingemarsson (1976)	0/15	0/15	
Larsen et al. (1986)	1/49	2/50	
Calder and Patel (1985)	0/37	1/39	
Scommegna (unpublished)	0/16	1/17	
Mariona (unpublished)	1/4	1/5	
Wesselius-De Casparis et al. (1971)	2/33	1/30	
Leveno et al. (1986)	2/56	3/55	
Larsen et al. (1980)	11/131	2/45	
Adam (1966)	9/28	7/24	
Typical odds ratio and 95% confidence interval			

Prostaglandin synthesis inhibitors (such as indomethacin) are effective but may have side effects in mother and fetus. Both β antagonists (ritodrine and salbutamol) and calcium antagonists (nifedipine) are used in the United Kingdom to suppress labour. These drugs work equally well on the myometrial cells and may postpone labour for a time. There is little evidence from meta-analyses of many studies that they reduce either perinatal mortality rates or postponement of labour over a long period.[2] Their use will depend on the ripeness of the cervix—the less ripe the more likely that action will be effective. They are best used before 32 weeks of pregnancy and probably work better in the absence of infection. Though little evidence shows that prophylactic oral β mimetic agents prevent preterm labour, oral maintenance after intravenous inhibition has some effect. Because of this, the recent introduction of oral nifedipine has been popular. The side effect profile is better, with occasional flushing, palpitations, and transient hypotension.

Once treatment with tocolytic agents has been started, the next decision is where the woman is to deliver if labour

Table 12.3 Effectiveness of β mimetic tocolytics used in preterm labour in reducing perinatal death. The numbers are the proportions of perinatal deaths[2]

Study	No in group		Odds ratio and 95% confidence interval
	Experimental	Control	0.01 0.1 0.5 1 2 10 100
Christensen et al. (1980)	14/14	16/16	
Spellacy et al. (1979)	12/14	13/15	
Barden (unpublished)	6/12	13/13	
Hoebel (unpublished)	10/16	8/15	
Cotton et al. (1984)	15/19	16/19	
Howard et al. (1982)	9/15	5/18	
Ingemarsson (1976)	3/15	12/15	
Larsen et al. (1986)	14/49	23/50	
Calder and Patel (1985)	23/37	19/39	
Scommegna (unpublished)	10/15	10/16	
Mariona (unpublished)	3/4	3/5	
Wesselius-De Casparis et al (1971)	13/33	21/30	
Leveno et al. (1986)	40/54	42/52	
Larsen et al. (1980)	65/131	21/45	
Sivasamboo (1972)	14/33	20/32	
Typical odds ratio and 95% confidence interval			

Note the small numbers and confidence intervals in some of the studies in this meta-analysis and the one on p. 75.

proceeds. If the unit cannot cope with very small babies, *in utero* transfer must be considered. The woman should go to a tertiary referral centre in the region that can manage babies of this degree of immaturity. The alternative philosophy is to allow the baby to be delivered in the peripheral centre and, if necessary, transfer the child to the tertiary referral unit by *ex utero* transfer. *In utero* transfer may not be necessary every time; it is used as a precaution but it allows the woman to be in the tertiary referral centre that is able to provide more sophisticated obstetric as well as neonatal care, for example Doppler flow studies. *Ex utero* transfer allows the woman to stay closer to her home at the local hospital she has chosen. However, specialist antenatal tests may not be available, obstetricians may not be as experienced in the delivery of very small babies, and expert paediatric teams may not be available at the time of delivery because of the many other calls on obstetricians' and paediatricians' time. In addition, with road traffic conditions in the UK there is no guarantee that help can get to even the nearest district hospital quickly. At present the

Box 12.3 Expert care for babies expected to be very small

- *In utero* transfer to obstetric/neonatal referral centre
- Delivery in district general hospital and *ex utero* transfer to specialist centre

philosophy is in favour of *in utero* transfer, but it may not stay so for long in the reorganised NHS.

Steroids, given to the mother before delivery, pass across the placenta to the fetus. Between 26 and 34 weeks' gestation, they have been shown to decrease morbidity and mortality associated with the respiratory immaturity of preterm delivery.[4] They are of optimal use if more than 24 hours passes from the first dose to delivery but often there is not enough time from the admission of the woman to her inevitable delivery. The use of tocolytic agents is used to postpone delivery and so extend the time available for the steroids to work on the fetal lung helping to produce surfactant. The steroids are commonly given as betamethasone in two intramuscular doses at 12-hour intervals. If labour is delayed by more than a week and the woman is still less than 34 weeks' gestation, the course of steroids is often repeated although the evidence of the benefits of this is hard to show.[5]

Conclusion

This and the previous chapter are concerned with the most serious problems of current obstetrics. Getting the best results for very small babies is the most hopeful line of advance at present. It needs coordination from family doctors, obstetricians, midwives, and neonatal paediatricians with individual treatments tailored to individual mothers.

The data for perinatal and neonatal mortality rates for Scotland are taken from the Scottish stillbirths and neonatal deaths report produced by the Information Office of the Scottish Health Service. The figure showing the cumulative distribution of singleton and multiple births is reproduced by permission of the Office of Population Censuses and Surveys from *Three, four and more*, published by HMSO. Other data come from CESDI reports.

Preterm labour and small for gestational age fetuses constitute the most serious current problems in obstetrics.

Reference

1 MacNaughton C, Chalmers T, Dubowitz V, *et al.* Report of the MRC/RCOG Multicentre randomised trial of cervical circlage. *Brit J Obstet Gynaec* 1993;**100**:516–20.
2 Chambers l, Enkin M, Keirse MJNC, eds. *Effective care in pregnancy and childbirth.* Vol 2. *Childbirth.* Oxford: Oxford University Press, 1989:705, 707.
3 McDonald H, Loughlin J, Jolley P, *et al.* Changes in vaginal flora during pregnancy and association with preterm birth. *J Infect Dis* 1994;**170**:724–8.
4 Crowley P, Chalmers I, Kierse M. The effects of cortical steroid administration before preterm delivery. *Br J Obstet Gynaec* 1990;**97**:11–25.
5 RCOG. *Antenatal corticosteroids to prevent respiratory disease syndrome.* RCOG Guideline No. 7 London: RCOG, 1996.

Recommended reading

● Chamberlain G. Antenatal care of the very small baby. In Harvey P, Cooke R, eds. *The baby under 1000 g.* Oxford: Butterworth Heinemann, 1999.
● Hyert J, Thilaganathan B. Obstetrics management at the limits of neonatal viability. In Studd J, ed. *Progress in obstetrics and gynaecology,* no. 14. London: Harcourt Brace, 2000.
● RCOG. *Antenatal corticosteroids to prevent respiratory distress syndrome. Guidelines no. 7.* London: RCOG, 1996.

13   Multiple pregnancy

Multiple pregnancy is a mixed blessing. On the one hand is the instant family, on the other are the increased perinatal mortality and morbidity as well as a much greater load for the mother after delivery.

Types

Multiple pregnancy follows either the division of an oocyte fertilised by one sperm into two separate bodies (identical or monozygotic twins) or the fertilisation of more than one egg by separate sperm (non-identical or dizygotic twins). In higher multiple pregnancies than twins a combination of these two mechanisms happens.

In monozygotic twins, division into two separate bodies was thought to occur only at a very early stage but it can in fact take place up to several days after fertilisation. The later this is, the more likely is the rare abnormality of conjoined twins.

Prevalence

The prevalence of twin births in the UK is 11.3/1000 deliveries, of triplets 0.3/1000, and of quadruplets about 0.01/1000 deliveries. There is a natural variation between races; Japanese women have one of the lowest rate of twins and those from some African countries have a much higher rate, up to one in 30 deliveries. Multiple pregnancies also increase with maternal age. These biological variations are due to an increase in the dizygotic twinning rates, based on the capacity of the woman to produce more than one oocyte at the time of ovulation.

The prevalence of multiple pregnancy has been increasing in the UK in the past decade. For higher multiples than twins the rate trebled from 12 per 100 000 to 40 per 100 000 between 1980 and 1998. Though a part of this is due to the increasing number of mothers over 35, the iatrogenic effect of ovarian stimulation and *in vitro* fertilisation programmes is also important. Concern about this led to the formation of a statutory body, the Human Fertilisation and Embryology Authority which made recommendations about the maximum number of oocytes or embryos transferred at assisted fertilisation, a limit of two.

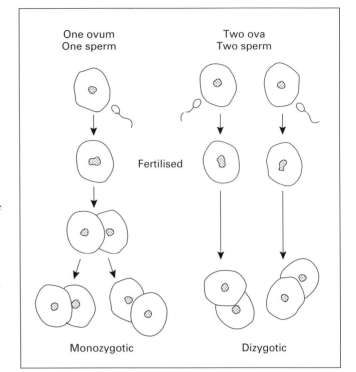

Figure 13.1 Monovular and binovular twins

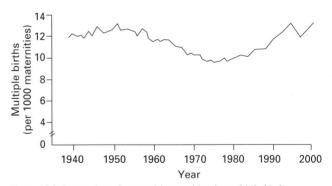

Figure 13.2 Proportion of maternities resulting in multiple births (England and Wales, 1939–98)

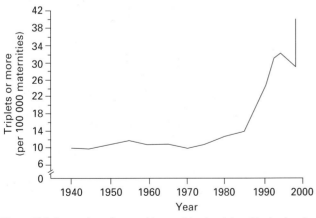

Figure 13.3 Proportion of maternities resulting in triplets (England and Wales, 1939–98)

Diagnosis

Twin pregnancies used to be diagnosed clinically when the woman reported her symptoms of pregnancy were worse than usual and the uterus was found to be bigger than would be

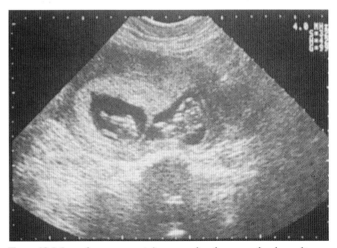

Figure 13.4 In early pregnancy twin sacs and embryos can be shown by ultrasonography

expected from gestational dates (after about 20 weeks); sometimes twins were diagnosed for the first time in labour. Often the fetal parts are hard to determine but palpation of more than two poles is suggestive of twins. Now in the UK most women have an ultrasound scan by 16 to 20 weeks and so multiple pregnancies are usually diagnosed much sooner. In the Scottish twin survey, 70% of multiple pregnancies were diagnosed by ultrasonography before 20 weeks and 95% in all were diagnosed in the antenatal period. The rest were diagnosed in labour. When a twin pregnancy is diagnosed by ultrasonography the increased incidence of congenital abnormalities should be remembered and a thorough ultrasound examination of each fetus performed between 20 and 24 weeks.

The increased uterine size leads to greater pressure on venous return. The frequency of the group of conditions that obstetricians (but not women) call minor problems (for example, varicose veins in the leg) is increased. Furthermore, the woman may have more symptoms of nausea in early pregnancy associated with the higher human chorionic gonadotrophin concentrations.

Death of one fetus

When one of a pair of twins dies *in utero* there is a risk to the mother of coagulopathy. For the surviving fetus there is also a risk of neurological lesions, preterm delivery with its problems of immaturity, and even intrauterine death. In very early pregnancy the complete absorption of the fetus that dies is usual (the vanishing twin phenomenon) probably happening in 5–8% of twin pregnancies. When fetal death comes later, it is best managed expectantly with close surveillance of the mother and the remaining fetus. In a dizygous twin pregnancy, the risks to the surviving fetus are relatively low.

One previously underconsidered feature of this problem has been the disaccord of the mother's reaction in grieving for one baby whilst looking forward hopefully to the birth of the other.

Congenital abnormalities

Many congenital abnormalities are more frequent in twins, especially those who are monozygous. Neural tube defects, heart abnormalities, and the incidences of Turner's and Klinefelter's syndromes are all increased. About twice as many live births from multiple pregnancies have a major congenital abnormality compared with singleton pregnancies.

Some of these abnormalities may be detected by ultrasound, others require amniocentesis. In multiple pregnancy this test is associated with a 3% rate of miscarriage compared with about 0.5% in singleton pregnancies. Care must be taken to identify the fluid from each sac, by proper labelling of the sample container, as the abnormality may be in one fetus only. Should severe abnormality be found in one fetus of a multiple pregnancy with two sacs the obstetrician may consider that the normal fetus is at increased risk and recommend selective fetocide. This can be by cardiac puncture, intravenous injection of potassium chloride or clipping the umbilical cord using a hysteroscope. Such management should be at a regional centre well used not just to performing these procedures but to the very important counselling that goes on before and after such an event. The risk of preterm labour in the unaffected pregnancy is increased.

Pregnancy-induced hypertension

The incidence of pregnancy-induced hypertension is increased in multiple pregnancies and eclampsia is also commoner. Antihypertensive treatment should be used as in any other pregnancy complicated by proteinuric hypertension

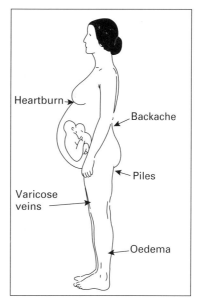

Figure 13.5 Changes that may follow an overdistended uterus with a multiple pregnancy

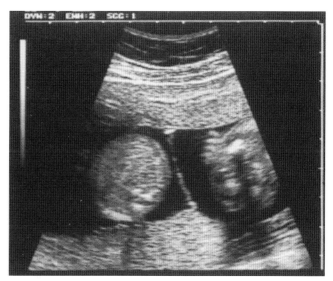

Figure 13.6 Twin fetuses at 16 weeks just before amniocentesis. Twin sacs are easily seen

(see Chapter 9), and the ultimate treatment of delivery may be required earlier than for singletons, a more difficult decision as preterm twin babies fare less well than do preterm singletons. A caesarean section is more frequently needed.

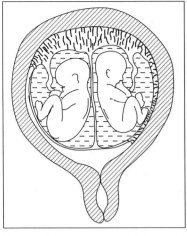

Figure 13.7 The greater area of placental implantation on the left of the uterus means that it may encroach on the lower segment

Anaemia

Commonly anaemia is reported as being more frequent in multiple than in singleton pregnancies. Some of this is due to the greater expansion in maternal blood volume with twins whereby the plasma increases more than the red cell bulk, so lowering the haemoglobin concentration. If the mean corpuscular haemoglobin concentration is used as a measure, anaemia is not more frequent in multiple pregnancies than in singletons provided that adequate nutrition and iron and folate intake are maintained. Greater demands of the growing fetuses for folate have led to some reports of megaloblastic anaemia, so folate supplements are commonly given.

Antepartum haemorrhage

Antepartum haemorrhage would be thought to be commoner in multiple pregnancy because of the greater surface area of the placental bed. The Aberdeen twin data set showed rates of antepartum haemorrhage in twin pregnancies to be 6% compared with 4.7% in singleton pregnancies ($p = <0.05$). Much of this difference, however, was made up of antepartum haemorrhage from unknown origin; only a few were caused by placental abruption or placenta praevia.

Intrauterine growth restriction

The growth of each fetus in multiple pregnancies mirrors that of the singleton until about 24 weeks of gestation; thence growth rates for most twins are still as for singletons but occasionally one or both may show a decrease. This is difficult to detect on clinical examination for polyhydramnios may cause imprecision in estimation of fetal size. Repeated serial ultrasound estimations of fetal size are the most useful way to check growth by plotting measurements of individual fetuses longitudinally through pregnancy. These data are not very different from the standard head or abdomen growth curves from singleton pregnancies until the last weeks. The estimation of fetal weight by various formulas based on the diameters of the fetus are not as useful in twin pregnancies as in the singleton.

Twin-to-twin transfusion

Twin-to-twin transfusion may be suspected when there is gross discordance in growth of a pair of twins or if there is

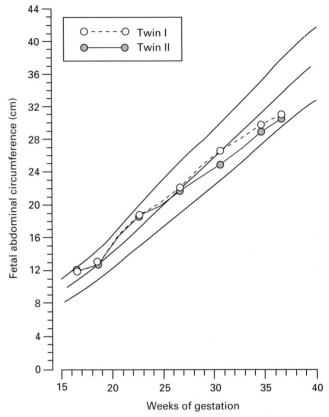

Figure 13.8 Growth of non-identical twins through pregnancy set against the mean (2 SD) singleton growth curve

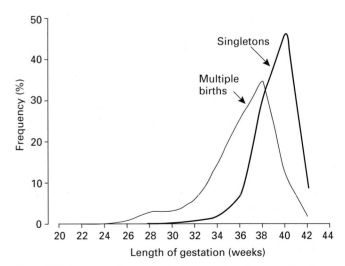

Figure 13.9 Percentage frequency distribution of length of gestation for singleton and twin pregnancies

polyhydramnios with one twin and oligohydramnios with the other. About 20% of monozygotic twin pregnancies have vascular connections between the two circulations inside the placenta but the imbalance of flow occurs in few of these, probably only 1% of such pregnancies. Clinical signs of stealing circulating blood from one twin by the other occurs less commonly and usually associated with a change in amniotic fluid volume which is quite obvious with ultrasound. If twins of the same sex are diagnosed by about 20 weeks gestation, careful ultrasound examination is made to determine chorionicity by assessing the number of discrete placental masses and the thickness of the membranes and their angle of approach to the decidual bed—the Lambda sign. While this warns of potential anastomoses, it is not of necessity grounds for fetocide, for sometimes the twin-to-twin transfusion can be compensated. It should lead to extra surveillance of both mother and fetus for the rest of the pregnancy.

Laser ablation of the communicating vessels of the placenta with intrauterine amnioscopes and narrow beam YAG laser is used; amnioreductions by amniocentesis may also be helpful.

Onset of preterm labour

The median gestation for human singleton pregnancy is just over 40 weeks whereas that for twins is 37 weeks and that for triplets about 33 weeks. The commonest single cause of perinatal mortality in multiple pregnancies is low birth weight. Though intrauterine growth restriction might also be present, birth weight is low mostly because of a preterm delivery. A measure of this problem is seen in the 30% of all liveborn triplets and 60% of liveborn quadruplets who have to stay in a neonatal intensive care unit for more than a month after delivery. The incidence of preterm labour (before 37 weeks) in twin pregnancies ranges from 20 to 50% compared with from 5 to 10% in singleton pregnancies.

An important part of antenatal care for multiple pregnancy is trying to detect those women who are likely to go into early preterm labour and prevent this if possible; if not, ensuring that they are delivered in the correct surroundings with neonatal unit facilities to look after immature babies. Some obstetricians find the examination of the cervix from 28 weeks gives a clue to its increasing ripeness (length, firmness, and dilatation). This seems to be of more use in primiparous than multiparous women. Others assess the cervix with ultrasound, endeavouring to predict early labour.

An essential element lies in informing the mother; antenatal education of women with twins about the signs of early preterm labour may be helpful.

The greater stretch of the myometrium imposed by multiple pregnancy increases the risk of preterm labour and several measures have been tried in the antenatal period to prevent this. Sympathomimetic drugs such as ritodrine have been given prophylactically, but most controlled trials have shown no benefit of this in twin pregnancy. Cervical cerclage inserted when a twin pregnancy is diagnosed does not seem to confer any increased benefits. Some consider that coitus may tip the balance in a woman who is on the edge of going into preterm labour, because of both the mechanical stimulation and the release into the vagina of prostaglandin-rich fluid. The avoidance of coitus in later pregnancy by women with twin pregnancies, however, does not seem to be associated with any significant prolongation of gestation.

Management

Antenatal care of a woman with a multiple pregnancy needs more vigilance than that of a woman with a singleton

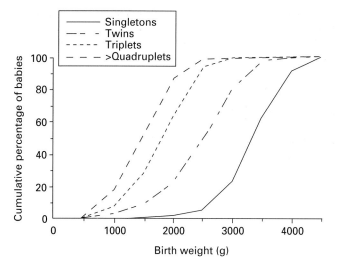

Figure 13.10 Birth weight distribution of singleton and multiple births

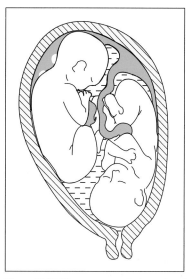

Figure 13.11 The extra stretch that twins place on the myometrium usually ensures that labour starts well before term

Box 13.1 Preparation of parents

- In pregnancy.
  - Why make frequent AN visits
  - When to give up outside work
  - Suitable diet for the mother
  - Potential delivery methods, e.g. CS
  - Visit to neonatal unit

- Discuss the future after twins are born.
  - Extra load for mother with two at once
  - Care of other children and husband
  - Help in home from relatives
  - Breast feeding
  - Local twins club
  - Is housing suitable?

pregnancy. The woman with a multiple pregnancy will need more social support and advice for she is embarking on an extra load before, during, and after delivery. Her socioeconomic state and its implications should be explored. She needs to be seen more often and will require more ultrasound investigations. Care can be shared with the general practitioner in early pregnancy but after about 24 weeks many obstetricians would prefer the care to be where tests can take place—the hospital antenatal clinic.

Antenatal diagnosis of fetal problems in multiple pregnancy must be preceded by careful counselling. All twins should have a detailed ultrasound scan for anomalies at 18–20 weeks and preferably a detailed fetal cardiac scan at 22–24 weeks. At least monthly ultrasound scans in the last trimester should be performed to monitor fetal growth.

Blood pressure and urinary protein concentration are checked at each clinic, as is the symphysio-fundal height. Palpation is performed by an experienced doctor or midwife.

Because of the increased risk of pregnancy-induced hypertension, women carrying twins were traditionally admitted to hospital from 32 weeks to ensure bedrest. The other justification for this was that it postponed preterm labour and so prolonged pregnancy. It is now realised that antenatal time in bed in hospital is not always the best rest: home is more relaxing. Furthermore, it would be more logical to bring the woman into hospital from 24 to 30 weeks, rather than at a later stage of pregnancy. Neither of the desirable aims has been fulfilled in randomised controlled trials of hospital admission after 32 weeks. Though reports from previous decades seemed to show a benefit in one or other of these aims (preventing raised blood pressure or postponing early labour), truly randomised studies in the 1990s have been unable to show benefit. When the disadvantages of separating the woman from her household, as well as the cost to society, are considered, the disadvantages of a routine policy of hospital admission outweigh the advantages. A woman should be advised, however, to come into hospital at a much lower critical level if, in her individual case, specific symptoms arise. These might include the development of hypertension or the threat of early preterm labour. The woman should be made well aware of the warning signs of preterm labour (see Chapter 12) and be encouraged to come in on a low level of suspicion.

Determination of the exact lie and presentation of each twin is often difficult in the last weeks of pregnancy. In many ways detail is not vital but the examiner should ensure that the leading twin is longitudinal. Nearly always the head or a breech is the lower presenting part. In cases of doubt a vaginal examination will usually give a clearer idea for if a presenting part is in or above the pelvis it can be identified more easily by the vaginal examination than through the abdominal wall. Ultrasonography will always confirm lie and presentation.

Delivery should be in a unit with experienced and sufficient staff to look after the resuscitation of both babies.

Many labours are complicated by the presence of one twin as a breech (up to 50%). Monitoring of each twin separately is necessary. An epidural anaesthetic provides good pain relief and less delay if operative delivery is needed quickly. A full account appears in *ABC of Labour*.

Outcome

Multiple pregnancies have increased risks for both mother and fetuses. Perinatal mortality rates are about four times higher among twins than singletons, being higher still among monozygotic twins. Rates are even greater in triplets and

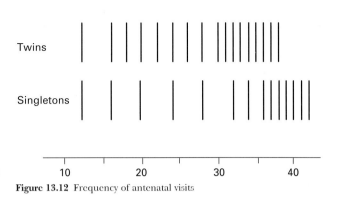

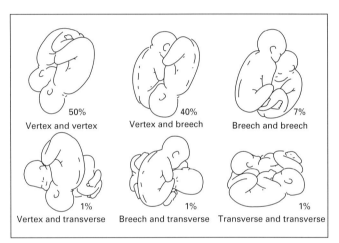

Figure 13.12 Frequency of antenatal visits

Box 13.2 Management of twin pregnancy
- Detailed ultrasound scan for abnormalities at 18–20 weeks
- Antenatal care at hospital clinic after 24 weeks
- More frequent antenatal visits
- Serial ultrasound scans to monitor fetal growth
- Watch for increased risk of maternal complications

Figure 13.13 Lie and presentation of twins at the start of labour

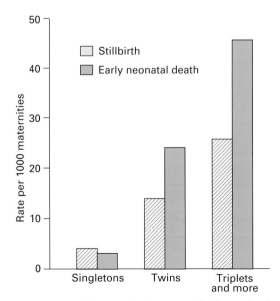

Figure 13.14 Still birth and early neonatal death rates for singleton and multiple pregnancies (England and Wales, 1998)

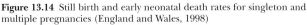

quadruplets. About three quarters of the increased mortality is caused by immaturity following preterm delivery, by intrauterine growth restriction or by some combination of the two. The perinatal mortality rate for the second twin at vaginal deliveries is much higher than that of the first, depending on the skills of the professional in charge of the delivery. The perinatal mortality rates associated with antepartum haemorrhage, premature rupture of the membranes, and proteinuric hypertension are increased.

Though some of the increased perinatal mortality rate in twins can be reduced by careful delivery, a large component can be helped by good antenatal care. This includes diagnosing the multiple pregnancy early, carefully managing the woman throughout pregnancy, and either postponing early preterm labour or if it must, ensuring that it takes place in an appropriate hospital with a good neonatal unit.

Triplets and more
With the increasing use of ovarian stimulation and other assorted fertility techniques, more women are becoming pregnant with higher multiples of fetus. All the complications that apply to twins can happen and more so. The risks are multiplied by the increased number; most triplets deliver before 35 weeks and usually by caesarean section. The survival to live birth of more than five fetuses is most unlikely and many doctors would advice fetal reduction down to two or three babies if the woman wishes this.

Recommended reading
- Botting B, MacFarlane A, Price F. *Three, four and more—a study of triplets and higher order births.* London: HMSO, 1990.
- Bryan E, Denton J, Hallet F. *Guidelines for professionals: multiple pregnancy.* London: Multiple Births Foundation, 1997.
- Ward R, Whittle M, eds. *Multiple pregnancy.* London: RCOG, 1995.
- Warner B, Keily J, Donovan E. Multiple births. *Clin Perinatol* 2000;**27**:347–61.

14   The audit of birth

Doctors are mostly literate but are commonly innumerate. We are largely ignorant and frightened of the safe and helpful use of figures because we have never been taught to understand them properly. We often try to dismiss them, believing that they are used during medical debate in a biased fashion to support the arguments of the proponents but are put to one side as non-relevant or non-significant by the opponents. This is a head in the sand attitude as statistics are extremely helpful in providing evidence of changes. Obstetricians should be well used to monitoring their activities statistically, having collected and published data long before the current fashion for audit started.

To be useful medical statistics must be:

- collected properly from a prescribed population;
- analysed in a valid fashion so as not to produce bias;
- presented promptly in a digestible, unbiased form.

Birth rates

The number of babies born is counted by two processes, birth registration and birth notification. These are two statutory obligations—registration by parents and notification by professional staff.

Birth rates are often expressed as a ratio of the number of births to the number of people in the existing population, gathered from the decennial census.

$$\text{Birth rate} = \frac{\text{No. of births} \times 1000}{\text{No. of people in the population}}$$

The birth rate in the UK in 1998 was 7.8 per 1000.

The denominator in this birth rate formula includes, however, men, who never give birth, and women under 15 and over 44, who are mostly outside the reproductive age group. Hence the denominator does not relate to the numerator very well; an alternative measure is more commonly used in the Western world:

$$\text{General fertility rate} = \frac{\text{No. of babies born} \times 1000}{\text{No. of women in the population aged 15--44}}$$

The general fertility rate in England and Wales in 1998 was 59 per 1000. International comparisons are harder because only countries with good census systems can break down population data to determine the number of women aged 15–44.

For the less numerically minded, completed family size is a user friendly statistic: we can all imagine the size of a family. Unfortunately, these data depend on uncertain estimates and are usually produced some years after the women concerned have passed their reproductive years and completed their family. Obviously, to increase any population the number in a family needs to be more than two. In much of western Europe it is 1.7 to 2.2, whereas in Kenya it is 6.9, showing a rapidly increasing population.

Perinatal mortality

Deaths of babies around the time of birth are assessed by three sets of statistics.

(1) Stillbirths or late intrauterine deaths occur when a child is delivered after the 24th completed week of pregnancy but shows no signs of life at birth:

$$\text{Stillbirth rate} = \frac{\text{No. of babies born dead after 24 weeks} \times 1000}{\text{Total births (live and stillborn)}}$$

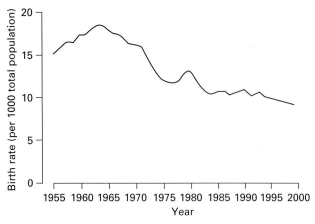

Figure 14.1 Birth rates in England and Wales, 1955–2000

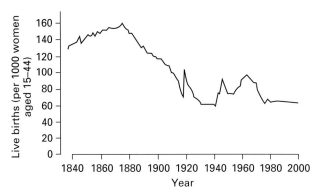

Figure 14.2 General fertility rates in England and Wales, 1840–2000

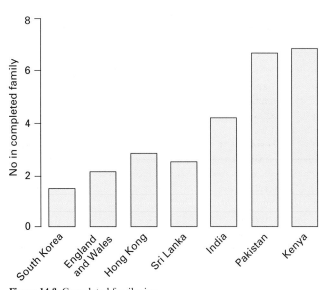

Figure 14.3 Completed family size

The stillbirth rate for England and Wales in 1998 was 5.3 per 1000 total births.

(2) Neonatal death is recorded when babies who are born alive (regardless of gestation) die in the first 28 days of life; early neonatal deaths refer to babies who die in the first seven days after birth. All babies who die in the first year of life are recorded as infant deaths but those who die after the first four weeks are defined as postneonatal deaths.

$$\text{Neonatal death rate} = \frac{\text{No. of babies dying between } 1\text{–}28 \text{ days} \times 1000}{\text{No. of live births}}$$

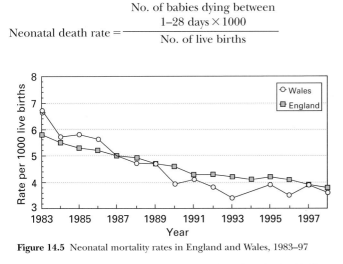

Figure 14.5 Neonatal mortality rates in England and Wales, 1983–97

The neonatal death rate for England and Wales in 1998 was 3.8 per 1000 live births.

(3) In the past 50 years perinatal mortality rates have been used to group together all babies whose deaths may have some relation to obstetric events; thus all stillbirths and neonatal deaths in the first week after birth are considered.

$$\text{Perinatal mortality rate} = \frac{\text{Stillbirths} + \text{neonatal deaths in the first 7 days} \times 1000}{\text{Total births (live and stillborn)}}$$

The perinatal mortality rate in England and Wales in 1998 was 7.9 per 1000 total births.

There is some degree of dissatisfaction with the use of perinatal mortality rates as an index of obstetric performance. Many babies born early now survive in neonatal units. Others with congenital lethal malformations may be kept alive in such units until the second or third week and so are not included in the perinatal mortality rate. We may return to looking at stillbirth rates and neonatal death rates as separate statistics. In 1992 in the UK, the gestation stage for viability was reduced from 28 to 24 weeks and so rates increased slightly around this time—a statistical but not a real blip.

The perinatal mortality rate has fallen steadily since the second world war. When data are compared from different countries, rates are falling in most of them at about the same rate, though some countries start worse off and stay there. This reflects the influence of socioeconomic factors and patterns of reproduction more than the quality of obstetric facilities. A similar pattern can be seen to a smaller extent in the regions of the UK.

The three main causes of perinatal mortality in the UK are low birth weight, hypoxia, and congenital abnormalities. Unfortunately, even after careful reexamination of notes and autopsy, some 70% of stillbirths are unexplained. Low birth weight is currently one of the biggest problems in the Western world (see Chapters 11 and 12). Hypoxia is mostly a problem of

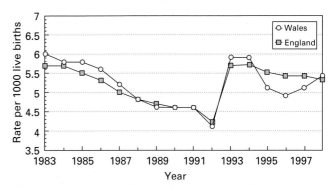

Figure 14.4 Stillbirth rates in England and Wales, 1983–97

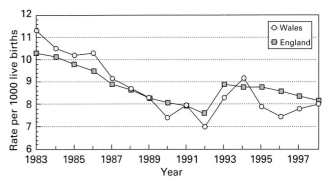

Figure 14.6 Perinatal mortality rates in England and Wales, 1983–97

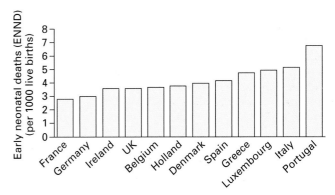

Figure 14.7 Early neonatal mortality rates (≤7 days) in the 12 countries of the then European community. (Source: Europe en Chiffers, Eurostat Office 1995)

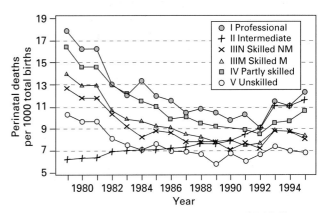

Figure 14.8 Perinatal mortality by father's social class 1979–95. (Source: ONS Mortality Statistics, DH3 series)

labour and to some extent is improved by monitoring women
at high risk. Congenital abnormalities may be detected at
antenatal examination (see Chapter 5) but the real cure of this
problem would be to prevent malformations rather than to
detect them and then abort the fetus.

Perinatal mortality rates are not a valid measure of obstetric
or midwifery performance. In a developed society they are a
mixed measure of a country's educational, social, nutritional,
and public health systems as well as of obstetric acute medicine.
The rate of deaths in the UK by socioeconomic class of the
father has narrowed over the years but still in 1995 PNMR of
Social Class I was 6.9 compared with 12.2 in Social Class V,
almost double. Probably only a third of the improvement in
perinatal mortality statistics is due to improvements in
medicine and midwifery. The rest is due to social and
economic factors.

A nationwide examination of stillbirths and neonatal deaths
together with infant deaths has now been developed, the
Confidential Enquiry into Stillbirths and Deaths in Infancy.
Reports are made to the regional centres and concentrated in
the Health Departments whence they are published each year.

Maternal mortality

Maternal deaths are rare in the Western world but this is not so
everywhere: in Kenya a woman has a chance as high as one in
20 of dying during one of her several pregnancies.

Maternal death usually refers to a woman dying in
pregnancy, childbirth, or within 42 days of the end of
pregnancy. In many countries, including the UK, it includes
deaths after an abortion or an ectopic pregnancy but in some
countries it does not. The definition in Britain used to include
deaths up to one year but has now come in line with World
Health Organisation recommendations.

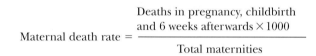

$$\text{Maternal death rate} = \frac{\substack{\text{Deaths in pregnancy, childbirth} \\ \text{and 6 weeks afterwards} \times 1000}}{\text{Total maternities}}$$

Maternal death rates in the UK did not reduce in this
century as swiftly as did the rates of perinatal death. Until the
mid-1930s maternal mortality was the same as it had been in
Victorian times. With the development of antibiotic therapy
the rates of puerperal sepsis reduced; to this was added the
improvements brought by a proper blood transfusion service
catalysed by the Second World War. The founding of the
colleges of midwives and obstetricians organised professional
training and standards, and the unification of the antenatal and
delivery services in the new NHS helped further.

International statistics on maternal mortality are less easy to
determine in a comparable way as different countries have
different exclusions. In general, however, maternal mortality is
an index of medical and midwifery care more than are the
perinatal mortality rates. Maternal death rates by region and by
country within the UK also vary but differently from perinatal
mortality rates.

In Britain the Confidential Enquiry into Maternal Deaths
has been set up to provide information about maternal deaths.
A complete case history of each maternal death is obtained and
published triennially by the Department of Health, keeping all
information confidential. The reports are published from the
whole UK rather than separately for the four kingdoms.

The maternal mortality in the UK was reported to be 7.4
per 100 000 in 1994–96; principal causes of maternal death in

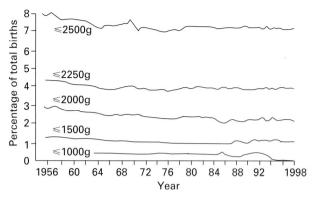

Figure 14.9 The proportions of babies in different birth weight bands
have altered little in the past 30 years

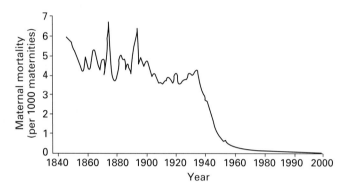

Figure 14.10 Maternal mortality in England and Wales, 1845–2000

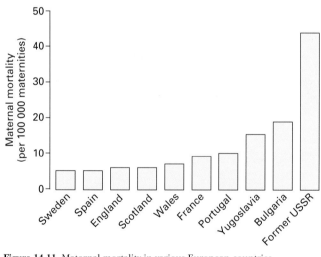

Figure 14.11 Maternal mortality in various European countries
(excluding deaths from abortion)

**Table 14.1 A total life risk assessment of maternal
deaths, derived from both the maternal mortality ratio
and the number of children a woman has (WHO 1996)**

Country	Risk
Norway	1 in 7300
Italy	1 in 5300
UK	1 in 5100
Australia	1 in 4900
USA	1 in 3500
Poland	1 in 2200
Cuba	1 in 490
China	1 in 400
Mexico	1 in 220
India	1 in 37
Zimbabwe	1 in 28
Kenya	1 in 20
Mali	1 in 10

England and Wales are hypertension and pulmonary embolism. To reduce the toll of hypertension the inquiry committee recommends that in each region there should be one or two hospitals with staff skilled at looking after pregnant hypertensive mothers and their fetuses. Women with severe degrees of this condition should be electively transferred to these centres. Pulmonary embolism commonly follows popliteal or pelvic vein thrombosis, which should be watched for, particularly in the puerperium after an operative delivery. An active policy of thromboprophylaxis could reduce this cause of death.

Other major killers in the past were infection and haemorrhage; currently these are much reduced. It must give satisfaction to those who fought for the Abortion Act of 1967 to find that in the last five triennia reported by the confidential inquiry committee (1982–96) there was not a single death from illegal abortion in England and Wales.

Near misses

An audit of serious complications such as haemorrhage over 1000 ml or pulmonary embolism in women who do not die gives an index of morbidity. Such near misses are harder to identify and collect but may be used in local audit. Definitions should be agreed and data collection should be prompt.

Conclusion

Too many doctors think of vital statistics in terms of Disraeli's, "Lies, damn lies and statistics".

Perhaps they should look at statistics in the same way as did Richard Asher: "When something can be expressed in a numerical way, it is an aid to precise and accurate thinking".

Most of the data in England and Wales are derived from the old Office of Population Censuses and Surveys, now the Office for National Statistics. The data on maternal mortality come from the Confidential Enquiries into Maternal Deaths for the UK and those of perinatal data from the Confidential Enquiry into Stillbirths and Deaths in Infancy for England and its parallel body in Wales.

Table 14.2   Major causes of maternal death (UK 1994–96)

		Rate per million maternities
Direct	Thromboembolism	21.8
	Hypertension	9.1
	Amniotic fluid embolism	7.7
	Haemorrhage	5.5
	Sepsis	6.4
	Anaesthesia	0.5
Indirect	Cardiac	16.4
	Psychiatric	4.1

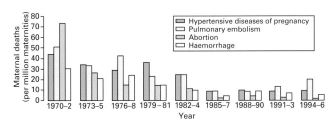

Figure 14.12 Major causes of maternal death in England and Wales, 1970–96

Recommended reading

- *Confidential enquiry into Stillbirths and Deaths in Infancy 1999.* London: ONS, 2000.
- Macfarlane A, Mugford M. *Birth counts.* London: Stationery Office, 2000.
- Office for National Statistics. *Why mothers die? Report on Confidential Enquiries into Maternal Deaths in the United Kingdom 1994–1996.* London: ONS, 1999.

L'envoi

Patterns of antenatal care shifted more in the last years of the 20th century than ever before. Less frequent visits for women with normal pregnancies and a wider sharing of professional responsibility are overtaking the hospital dominated and regimented patterns of the middle of the last century.

The development of antenatal care reflects what has happened in all of medicine—first came the clinical observations, then the mounting of investigations, each supported by some scientific pedigree, and only later a guilty sideways look at what value these all provided. In an ideal world all the investigations would have been subjected to rigorous scrutiny—randomised controlled trials and careful checks of sensitivity and specificity—but such intellectual disciplines were introduced after many of the antenatal tests had been started. We did not await the more scientifically assessed investigation because babies were still being born and women still needed to know. Meanwhile, we do the best with what we have. Clinical management should reflect the results of research studies and must depend in future more upon evidence based research promptly delivered.

If we were to see women in appropriate circumstances and make proper use of the proven valuable tests we already have, much effort and money would be saved. We could spend more time listening to and talking with the women we care for. The golden age of antenatal care would then have arrived.

Index

Page numbers in **bold** type refer to figures; those in italic refer to tables or boxed material

Index

Index